CUTANEOUS CONDITION INTRODUCTION

Books LLC®, Reference Series, Memphis, USA, 2011. ISBN: 9781151022714. www.booksllc.net.

Table of Contents

Introduction

Purchase of this book entitles you to a free trial membership in the publisher's book club at www.booksllc.net. (Time limited offer.) Simply enter the barcode number from the back cover onto the membership form. The book club entitles you to select from hundreds of thousands of books at no additional charge. You can also download a digital copy of this and related books to read on the go. Simply enter the title or subject onto the search form to find them.

Each chapter in this book ends with a URL to a hyperlinked online version. Type the URL exactly as it appears. If you change the URL's capitalization it won't work. Use the online version to access related pages, websites, footnotes, tables, color photos, updates. Click the version history tab to see the chapter's contributors. Click the edit link to suggest changes.

A large and diverse editor base collaboratively wrote the book, not a single author. After a long process of discussion and debate, the chapters gradually took on a neutral point of view reached through consensus. Additional editors expanded and contributed to chapters striving to achieve balance and comprehensive coverage. This reduced the regional or cultural bias found in many other books and provided access and breadth on subject matter otherwise little documented.

ANOTHER syndrome

ANOTHER syndrome consists of alopecia, nail dystrophy, ophthalmic complications, thyroid dysfunction, hypohidrosis, ephelides and enteropathy, and respiratory tract infections. This is an autosomal recessive variant of ectodermal dysplasia.

Source (edited): "http://en.wikipedia.org/wiki/ANOTHER_syndrome"

Abietic acid dermatitis

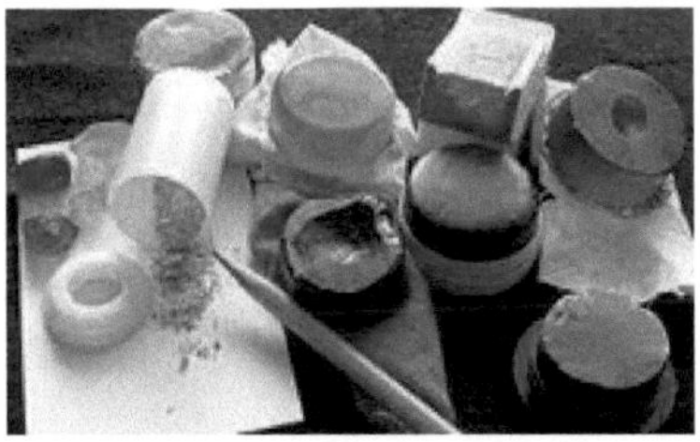

Various types of rosin for violins, violas and cellos

Abietic acid dermatitis is a contact dermatitis often seen in association with musical instruments.

Causes

The main cause is a a type-I hypersensitivity reaction to products containing abietic acid, such as the Rosin/colophony, which is commonly used as a friction-increasing agent. Players of bowed string instruments (Violin, viola, cello, double bass) rub cakes or blocks of rosin on their bow so it can grip the strings. Ballet and flamenco dancers sometimes rub their shoes in powdered rosin to reduce slippage before going on stage. Gymnasts, Baseball pitchers and ten pin bowlers also use rosin to improve grip. The common locations of this contact dermatitis are: Hands, face and neck

Differential diagnosis

Cutaneous disorders in musicians include frictional injury ("fiddler's neck"), hyperhidrosis, acne mechanica and vascular compromise. Other agents of irritant and allergic contact dermatitis may be: Rosewood, Makassar Ebony, Cocobolo wood, African blackwood, Nickel, Reed, Propolis (bee glue), Chromium and Paraphenylenediamine. Patch testing can be performed for identification of the cause.

Treatment

Treatment may include corticoids, astringents and keratolytics. Dermatoses tend to be recurrent unless the use or contact can be avoided. Discontinuation of the instrument is curative in almost all cases, but usually quite impractical.

Source (edited): "http://en.wikipedia.org/wiki/Abietic_acid_dermatitis"

Acanthosis nigricans associated with malignancy

Acanthosis nigricans associated with malignancy (also known as "Acanthosis nigricans type I") is the "malignant" type of acanthosis nigricans that may either precede (18%), accompany (60%), or follow (22%) the onset of an internal cancer. Malignancy-associated acanthosis nigricans is usually rapid in onset and may be accompanied by skin tags, multiple seborrheic keratoses, or tripe palms.

Source (edited): "http://en.wikipedia.org/wiki/Acanthosis_nigricans_associated_with_malignancy"

Acanthosis nigricans associated with obesity, insulin-resistant states, and endocrinopathy

Acanthosis nigricans associated with obesity, insulin-resistant states, and endocrinopathy (also known as "Acanthosis nigricans type III") is the most common variety of acanthosis nigricans, presenting with a grayish, velvety thickening of the skin on the sides of the neck, axillae, and groins. Acanthosis nigricans associated with endocrine dysfunction is more insidious in its onset, is less widespread, and the patients are often obese.

Source (edited): "http://en.wikipedia.org/wiki/Acanthosis_nigricans_associated_with_obesity,_insulin-resistant_states,_and_endocrinopathy"

Acne aestivalis

Acne aestivalis (also known as **Mallorca acne**) is a special form of polymorphous light eruption. It is a monomorphous eruption consisting of multiple, uniform, red, papular lesions, reported to occur after sun exposure.

Source (edited): "http://en.wikipedia.org/wiki/Acne_aestivalis"

Acne cosmetica

Acne cosmetica is a term referring to acne caused by or made worse by cosmetics. The mechanism was presumably a chemically induced plugging of the pilosebaceous orifice. This was a significant problem for dermatologists in the 1970s and 1980s, but with the improved formulations produced by cosmetic chemists over the past thirty years, this is now a relatively rare diagnosis in daily practice.

The terms "non-comedogenic" and "non-acne(i)genic" appeared on moisturizers and other cosmetic compounds as re-formulations were introduced, sometimes associated with claims that the products were oil-free or water-based. Although early work produced lists of comedogenic chemicals in various strengths and vehicles, it became apparent that the actual comedogenicity of a product could not be predicted from its contents; rather the finished product itself needed to be use-tested.

The production of a low-grade folliculitis by some components of cosmetic products has led to misdiagnosis on occasion.

People may not attribute their reactions to their cosmetics at first, but may notice worsening symptoms after using certain face makeup, sunblock or lip products.

Reactions are more likely to occur if applied cosmetics are let to sit and are not stripped after use.

Source (edited): "http://en.wikipedia.org/wiki/Acne_cosmetica"

Acne fulminans

Acne fulminans (also known as "Acute febrile ulcerative acne") is a severe form of the skin disease, acne, which can occur after unsuccessful treatment for another form of acne, acne conglobata. The condition is thought to be an immunologically induced disease in which elevated level of testosterone causes a rise in sebum and P acne bacterias. The condition is commonly, albeit inefficiently treated with steroids.

Symptoms

Acne fulminans begins as pain and inflammation in the joints. It eventually progresses into a swelling of the lymph nodes located at the base of the neck, causing inflexibility in the neck within weeks after the nodes swell. This swelling will eventually decrease, but this decrease will be accompanied by an increased inflammation and swelling of the joints, as well as a complete loss of appetite, though these symptoms are often ignored. After some time, the disease will cause an extreme loss of weight and atrophy of the muscles, leading to the decline of physical abilities.

Treatment

Treatment should be sought immediately in order to avoid hospitalization. If not treated, hospitalization for an extended period of time (usually two weeks) is likely. During hospitalization, the patient is tested for signs of system degradation, especially of the skeletal structure and the digestive tract. By this time open sores will develop on the upper torso. Some will be the size of dimes, others will be large enough to stick a couple fingers into. They will crust up, causing cohesion to any fabric the sores touch, which is extremely painful to remove. It is recommended to sleep on ones sides until the cystic condition subsides, in order to avoid any uncomfortable situations. Once inflammation goes down, one should resume sleeping on one's front or back, to avoid any complications with shoulder issues in the future (such as spontaneous dislocation).

The disease activates at the height of puberty, usually at around 13 years of age.

Source (edited): "http://en.wikipedia.org/wiki/Acne_fulminans"

Acne keloidalis nuchae

Acne keloidalis nuchae (also known as "Acne keloidalis", "Dermatitis papillaris capillitii", "Folliculitis keloidalis", "Folliculitis keloidis nuchae", and "Nuchal keloid acne") is a destructive scarring folliculitis that occurs almost exclusively on the occipital scalp of people of African descent, primarily men. This is mainly because men often cut their hair very low as opposed to women, allowing the hair to prick the occipital scalp and upset it. Acne keloidalis nuchae most commonly presents itself in individuals aged 13 to 25.

Source (edited): "http://en.wikipedia.org/wiki/Acne_keloidalis_nuchae"

Acne mechanica

Acne mechanica is an acneiform eruption that has been observed after repetitive physical trauma to the skin such as rubbing, occurring from clothing (belts and straps) or sports equipment (football helmets and shoulder pads).

Source (edited): "http://en.wikipedia.org/wiki/Acne_mechanica"

Acne medicamentosa

Acne medicamentosa (commonly referred to as **drug-induced acne**) is acne that is caused or aggravated by medication. Because acne is generally a disorder of the pilosebaceous units caused by hormones, the medications that trigger acne medicamentosa most frequently are hormone analogues. It is also often caused by corticosteroids; in this case, it is referred to as steroid acne.

Although the masculinizing hormone testosterone is most often blamed, and although men with acne secondary to bodybuilding hormones are seen from time to time, the major hormonal medications that causes acne are the progestin analogues present in hormonal contraception. Other medications can produce acneiform eruptions (usually pimply bumps and pustules that look like acne).

Some conditions mimic acne medicamentosa. The most common mimic is folliculitis produced by an overgrowth of the *Malassezia* species, often secondary to oral or systemic corticosteroids, or secondary to broad-spectrum antibiotics such as the tetracycline family used in acne. This is often misinterpreted as 'tetracycline-resistant acne'.

Source (edited): "http://en.wikipedia.org/wiki/Acne_medicamentosa"

Acne miliaris necrotica

Acne miliaris necrotica (also known as "Acne varioliformis") consists of follicular vesicopustules, sometimes occurring as solitary lesions that are usually very itchy.

Source (edited): "http://en.wikipedia.org/wiki/Acne_miliaris_necrotica"

Acne with facial edema

Acne with facial edema (also known as "Solid facial edema") occurs uncommonly, and is associated with a peculiar inflammatory edema of the mid-third of the face.

Source (edited): "http://en.wikipedia.org/wiki/Acne_with_facial_edema"

Acquired C1 esterase inhibitor deficiency

Acquired C1 esterase inhibitor deficiency presents with symptoms indistinguishable from hereditary angioedema, but generally with onset after the fourth decade of life.

C4 levels are low and C3 levels are normal.

Source (edited): "http://en.wikipedia.org/wiki/Acquired_C1_esterase_inhibitor_deficiency"

Acquired dyskeratotic leukoplakia

Acquired dyskeratotic leukoplakia is a condition characterized by distinctive white plaques on the palate, gingivae, and lips.

Source (edited): "http://en.wikipedia.org/wiki/Acquired_dyskeratotic_leukoplakia"

Acquired generalized lipodystrophy

Acquired generalized lipodystrophy (also known as "Lawrence syndrome," and "Lawrence–Seip syndrome") is a rare skin condition that appears during childhood or adolescence, characterized by fat loss affecting large areas of the body, particularly the face, arms, and legs.

Source (edited): "http://en.wikipedia.org/wiki/Acquired_generalized_lipodystrophy"

Acral acanthosis nigricans

Acral Acanthosis Nigricans also known as **Acral Acanthotic Anomaly (AAA)** - Acral acanthosis nigricans is a common and thus important variant of Acanthosis nigricans. Classical acanthosis nigricans is characterized by hyperpigmented, velvety thickening of the skin typically on the nape and sides of the neck and in the axillae and groin . It is also known as acral acanthotic anomaly, the two terms being synonymous. The former emphasizes that it is a type of acanthosis nigricans, the latter its uniqueness. It was discovered by internationally renowned dermatologist Robert A. Schwartz. Its original description in 1981 observed it as a disorder seen relatively commonly as velvety hyperpigmented plaques in dark complexioned individuals. It is often particularly prominent over the elbows, knees, knuckles and dorsal surfaces of the feet in otherwise healthy individuals with axillae and other intertriginous regions appearing normal.

Etiology

The etiology of acral acanthosis nigricans is unknown. Its presence does not suggest the necessary of an evaluation for the presence of internal malignancy.

Source (edited): "http://en.wikipedia.org/wiki/Acral_acanthosis_nigricans"

Acral dry gangrene

Acral dry gangrene is a cutaneous condition characterized by necrosis of the fingertips or toes and may be associated with diabetes mellitus.

Source (edited): "http://en.wikipedia.org/wiki/Acral_dry_gangrene"

Acral nevus

An **Acral nevus** (also known as a "**Melanocytic nevus of acral skin**", and "**Melanocytic nevus with intraepidermal ascent of cells**" (**MANIACS**)) is a cutaneous condition characterized by a skin lesion that is usually macular or only slightly elevated, and may display uniform brown or dark brown color, but often with linear striations.

Source (edited): "http://en.wikipedia.org/wiki/Acral_nevus"

Acral persistent papular mucinosis

Acral persistent papular mucinosis is a skin condition caused by fibroblasts producing abnormally large amounts of mucopolysaccharides, characterized by bilaterally symmetrical, flesh-colored papules localized to the hands and wrists.

Source (edited): "http://en.wikipedia.org/wiki/Acral_persistent_papular_mucinosis"

Acroangiodermatitis

Acroangiodermatitis of Mali (also known as "Mali acroangiodermatitis" and "Pseudo-Kaposi's sarcoma") is a rare cutaneous condition often characterized by purplish-blue to brown papules and plaques on the medial and lateral malleolus of both legs.

Acroangiodermatitis is a rare skin condition characterised by hyperplasia of pre-existing vasculature due to venous hypertension from severe chronic venous stasis. It is associated with amputees, haemodialysis (HD) patients with arteriovenous (AV) shunts, and patients with paralysed legs, hepatitis C, chronic venous insufficiency or AV malformations (AVM). Patients present with itchy, painful, confluent, violaceous or brown-black macules, papules or plaques usually at the distal lower limbs. There may be ulceration and bleeding. The histologic features are capillary proliferation and perivascular inflammation involving eosinophils in the dermis with minimal epidermal changes. Management includes compression therapy, wound care and surgical correction of AVM. Dapsone combined with leg elevation and compression, and erythromycin for HD patients with AV fistulas have also been reported. The lesions may persist for years with complications like ulceration, bleeding and infection.

Source (edited): "http://en.wikipedia.org/wiki/Acroangiodermatitis"

Acrokeratoelastoidosis of Costa

Acrokeratoelastoidosis of Costa (also known as "Keratoelastoidosis marginalis") is a familial condition characterized by multiple keratotic papules on the dorsum of the hands and feet, palms, soles, in which electron microscopy shows rarified, abnormal elastic tissue.

It was characterized in 1953.

Treatments such as liquid nitrogen, salicylic acid, tretinoin, and prednisone have been tried, though with limited success.

Source (edited): "http://en.wikipedia.org/wiki/Acrokeratoelastoidosis_of_Costa"

Actinic granuloma

Actinic granuloma (also known as "O'Brien granuloma") is a cutaneous condition characterized histologically by a dermal infiltrate of macrophages.

Source (edited): "http://en.wikipedia.org/wiki/Actinic_granuloma"

Actinic prurigo

Actinic prurigo (also known as "Familial polymorphous light eruption of American Indians," "Hereditary polymorphous light eruption of American Indians," "Hutchinson's summer prurigo," and "Hydroa aestivale") is a not uncommon sunlight-induced, pruritic, papular or nodular skin eruption.

History

Actinic prurigo (AP) was first described by Escalona in Mexico, in 1954.

Causes

The cause for actinic prurigo is unknown, however researchers believe that the protein in our bodies may be a cause to the condition also: •UV-A and UV-B light seem to be the main provoking agents. This observation is supported by the fact that most patients live at high altitudes (>1000 m above sea level), and the condition improves in many patients when they move to lower altitudes. However, some patients who are affected already live at sea level.18,19,27 •Some authors are considering a food photosensitizer or a nutritional selective deficiency as a cause; however, no evidence proves this theory.27

Symptoms

AP is characterized by itchy, inflamed papules, nodules, and plaques on the skin. Lesions typically appear hours or days after exposure of the skin to UV light, and follow a general pattern of sun-exposed areas. The face, neck, arms, hands, and legs are often affected, although lesions sometimes appear on skin that is covered by clothing and thus not exposed to UV light, thus making AP somewhat difficult to diagnose.

AP is a chronic disease, and symptoms usually worsen in the spring and summer as the day lengthens and exposure to sunlight increases.

Treatment

Currently there is no cure for actinic prurigo, and treatment focuses on relieving the dermatologic symptoms, by way of topical steroid creams or systemic immunosuppressants.

Prescribed treatments include:

- topical creams such as Tacrolimus and Betamethasone.
- systemic immunosuppressants such as Prednisone.
- In some cases, Thalidomide has proven to be effective in controlling the symptoms of actinic prurigo.

All patients with AP are encouraged to

minimize sun exposure, and to use strong sunscreen throughout the year, and even on cloudy or overcast days, as UVA light, unlike UVB light, is able to penetrate cloud cover and remains constant throughout the day.

Alternative treatment methods might include UV Hardening, Meditation and/ or cognitive behavioral therapy. The U. S. Food and Drug Administration (FDA) has yet to approve these allopathic approaches to medicine, so there remains much to be discovered about this particular illness in the United States.

Source (edited): "http://en.wikipedia.org/wiki/Actinic_prurigo"

Acute erythema nodosum

Acute erythema nodosum is a skin condition, a reactive process commonly associated with a streptococcal infection which, in children, is by far the most common precipitant.

Source (edited): "http://en.wikipedia.org/wiki/Acute_erythema_nodosum"

Acute generalized exanthematous pustulosis

Acute generalized exanthematous pustulosis (AGEP) (also known as "Pustular drug eruption," and "Toxic pustuloderma") is a not uncommon cutaneous reaction pattern that in 90% of cases is related to medication administration, characterized by a sudden eruption that appears on average five days after the medication is started.

It is mediated by T cells.

Presentation

AGEP is an acute febrile drug eruption characterized by numerous small, primarily non-follicular, sterile pustules, arising within large areas of edematous erythema.

The eruption follows a self-limiting course and will end before a week provided the causative agent (e.g. medication) is discarded. It is accompanied by fever, neutrophilia, and sometimes by facial edema, hepatitis and eosinophilia. The mortality rate is about 5% and the differential diagnosis must include the dreaded Stevens-Johnson syndrome (SJS). Contrary to SJS, in AGEP, mucosa are not affected, which means that there are no blisters in the mouth or vagina.

Treatment

The treatment is (1) stop the offending drug (antibiotics), (2) symptomatic (fever) and (3) for complications (hepatitis).

Source (edited): "http://en.wikipedia.org/wiki/Acute_generalized_exanthematous_pustulosis"

Acute hemorrhagic edema of infancy

Acute hemorrhagic edema of infancy (also known as "Acute hemorrhagic edema of childhood," "Finkelstein's disease," "Infantile postinfectious iris-like purpura and edema," "Medallion-like purpura," "Purpura en cocarde avec oedema," and "Seidlmayer syndrome") is a skin condition that affects children under the age of two with a recent history of upper respiratory illness, a course of antibiotics, or both.

Source (edited): "http://en.wikipedia.org/wiki/Acute_hemorrhagic_edema_of_infancy"

Acute radiodermatitis

Acute radiodermatitis occurs when an "erythema dose" of ionizing radiation is given to the skin, after which visible erythema appears up to 24hrs after. Radiation dermatitis generally manifests within a few weeks after the start of radiotherapy. Acute radiodermatitis, while presenting as red patches, may sometimes also present with desquamation or blistering. Erythema may occur at a dose of 2 Gy radiation or greater.

Source (edited): "http://en.wikipedia.org/wiki/Acute_radiodermatitis"

Acute urticaria

Acute urticaria is defined as the presence of evanescent wheals which completely resolve within six weeks.

Acute urticaria becomes evident a few minutes after the person has been exposed to the allergen. The outbreak of acute urticaria may last several weeks, but usually the hives are gone in six weeks. Typically, the hives are a reaction to food but in half the causes the trigger is unknown. Common foods may be the cause, as well as bee or wasp stings, or skin contact with certain fragrances.

Source (edited): "http://en.wikipedia.

org/wiki/Acute_urticaria"

Adrenergic urticaria

Adrenergic urticaria is a skin condition characterized by an eruption consisting of small (1-5mm) red macules and papules with a pale halo, appearing within 10 to 15 min after emotional upset.

Source (edited): "http://en.wikipedia.org/wiki/Adrenergic_urticaria"

Adult blaschkitis

Adult blaschkitis is a rare inflammatory skin condition presenting as pruritic papules and vesicles along multiple lines of Blaschko.

Source (edited): "http://en.wikipedia.org/wiki/Adult_blaschkitis"

Adult linear IgA disease

Adult linear IgA disease is an acquired, autoimmune blistering disease that may present with a clinical pattern of vesicles indistinguishable from dermatitis herpetiformis, or with vesicles and bullae in a bullous pemphigoid-like appearance.

Source (edited): "http://en.wikipedia.org/wiki/Adult_linear_IgA_disease"

Adverse reaction to biologic agents

Adverse reactions to biologic agents, such as imatinib, occur in more than 80% of patients, and can be characterized by edema and pruritus without dermatitis.

Source (edited): "http://en.wikipedia.org/wiki/Adverse_reaction_to_biologic_agents"

Adverse reaction to cytokines

Adverse reactions to cytokines are characterized by local inflammation and/or ulceration at the injection sites, and occasional present with more widespread papular eruptions.

Source (edited): "http://en.wikipedia.org/wiki/Adverse_reaction_to_cytokines"

African blackwood dermatitis

African blackwood dermatitis is a condition characterized by an allergic contact dermatitis associated with a musical instrument made of a particular type of wood.

Source (edited): "http://en.wikipedia.org/wiki/African_blackwood_dermatitis"

Airbag dermatitis

Airbag dermatitis (also known as an "Airbag burn") is caused skin irritation and trauma secondary to the deployment of airbags.

Source (edited): "http://en.wikipedia.org/wiki/Airbag_dermatitis"

Albinism–deafness syndrome

Albinism–deafness syndrome (also known as "Woolf syndrome," and "Ziprkowski–Margolis syndrome") is a condition characterized by congenital neural deafness and a severe or extreme piebald-like phenotype with extensive areas of hypopigmentation.

A locus at Xq26.3-q27.I has been suggested.

It has been suggested that it is a form of Waardenburg syndrome type II.

Source (edited): "http://en.wikipedia.org/wiki/Albinism%E2%80%93deafness_syndrome"

Alezzandrini syndrome

Alezzandrini syndrome is a very rare syndrome characterized by a unilateral degenerative retinitis, followed after several months by ipsilateral vitiligo on the face and ipsilateral poliosis. Deafness may also be present.

Source (edited): "http://en.wikipedia.org/wiki/Alezzandrini_syndrome"

Allergic contact cheilitis

Allergic contact cheilitis is a conditions of the lips characterized by a dryness, fissuring, edema, and crusting.

Source (edited): "http://en.wikipedia.org/wiki/Allergic_contact_cheilitis"

Allopurinol hypersensitivity syndrome

Allopurinol hypersensitivity syndrome typically occurs in persons with preexisting renal failure. Weeks to months after allopurinol is begun, the patient develops a morbilliform eruption.

Source (edited): "http://en.wikipedia.org/wiki/Allopurinol_hypersensitivity_syndrome"

Alpha-1 antitrypsin deficiency panniculitis

Alpha-1 antitrypsin deficiency panniculitis (also known as "Alpha1-protease deficiency panniculitis," and "Alpha1-proteinase deficiency panniculitis") is a skin condition characterized by inflammation of the subcutaneous fat associated with a deficiency of the α-antitrypsin enzyme.

Source (edited): "http://en.wikipedia.org/wiki/Alpha-1_antitrypsin_deficiency_panniculitis"

Amelanotic blue nevus

An **Amelanotic blue nevus** (also known as a "Hypomelanotic blue nevus") is a cutaneous condition characterized by mild atypia and pleomorphism.

Source (edited): "http://en.wikipedia.org/wiki/Amelanotic_blue_nevus"

Amelanotic melanoma

Amelanotic melanoma is a type of skin cancer in which the cells do not make melanin.

Source (edited): "http://en.wikipedia.org/wiki/Amelanotic_melanoma"

Androgen-dependent syndromes

Androgen-dependent syndromes are caused by the excessive production of adrenal or gonadal androgens by adrenal adenomas, carcinomas, or hyperplasia, Leydig cell tumors in men, and arrhenoblastomas and polycystic ovarian syndrome in women.

Source (edited): "http://en.wikipedia.org/wiki/Androgen-dependent_syndromes"

Anetoderma

Anetoderma (also known as "Anetoderma maculosa," "Anetoderma maculosa cutis," "Atrophia maculosa cutis," and "Macular atrophy") is a localized laxity of the skin with herniation or outpouching resulting from abnormal dermal elastic tissue.

Source (edited): "http://en.wikipedia.org/wiki/Anetoderma"

Angina bullosa haemorrhagica

Angina bullosa haemorrhagica is a condition of the mucous membranes characterized by the sudden appearance of one or more blood blisters within the oral cavity. The lesions, which may be caused by mild trauma to the mouth tissues such as hot foods, typically rupture quickly and heal without scarring or further discomfort. The condition is not serious except in rare cases where a large bulla that does not rupture spontaneously may cause airway obstruction.

The blisters usually affect the palate or oropharynx and are often long lived to the extent that patients burst them for symptomatic relief.

Diagnosis

The conidtion is diagnosed on the basis of exclusion of other conditions and the typical presentation, particularly the constant presence of blood as the blister fluid. Angina bullosa haemorrhagica does not cause desquamative gingivitis
Source (edited): "http://en.wikipedia.org/wiki/Angina_bullosa_haemorrhagica"

Angiocentric lymphoma

Angiocentric lymphoma (also known as "Extranodal natural killer cell lymphoma," "Nasal-type NK lymphoma," "NK/T-cell lymphoma," and "Polymorphic/malignant midline reticulosis") is a cutaneous condition which in Korea, is reported to be the most common form of cutaneous lymphoma after mycosis fungoides.

Extranodal NK-T-cell lymphoma is a type of lymphoma.

It is called "extranodal" to emphasize that the location is not in the lymph node. It is sometimes further qualified as "nasal type".

It can be associated with Epstein Barr virus.
Source (edited): "http://en.wikipedia.org/wiki/Angiocentric_lymphoma"

Annular elastolytic giant-cell granuloma

Annular elastolytic giant-cell granuloma (also known as "Giant cell elastophagocytosis," "Meischer's granuloma," "Miescher's granuloma of the face") is a cutaneous condition characterized histologically by a dermal infiltrate of macrophages.
Source (edited): "http://en.wikipedia.org/wiki/Annular_elastolytic_giant-cell_granuloma"

Annular lichen planus

Annular lichen planus occurs in approximately ten percent of lichen planus cases, and commonly develop as arcuate groupings of individual papules that develop rings or peripheral extension of clustered papules with central clearing.
Source (edited): "http://en.wikipedia.org/wiki/Annular_lichen_planus"

Annular pustular psoriasis

Annular pustular psoriasis is a rare variant of pustular psoriasis, having an annular, or circinate, lesion morphology that may appear at the onset of pustular psoriasis, with a tendency to spread and form enlarged rings.
Source (edited): "http://en.wikipedia.org/wiki/Annular_pustular_psoriasis"

Annular sarcoidosis

Annular sarcoidosis is a cutaneous condition characterized by papular skin lesions arranged in annular patterns, usually with a red-brown hue.
Source (edited): "http://en.wikipedia.org/wiki/Annular_sarcoidosis"

Anticoagulant-induced skin necrosis

Anticoagulant-induced skin necrosis can be caused by both warfarin and heparin. Though by different mechanism, obese, postmenopausal woman have a predisposition. Skin lesions tend to occur in areas with abundant subcuta-

neous fat such as the breast, abdomen, and buttocks. Warfarin necrosis occurs three to five days after therapy is begun, and a high initial dose increases risk. Heparin induced necrosis both at sites of local injection and in a widespread pattern when infused intravenously.
Source (edited): "http://en.wikipedia.org/wiki/Anticoagulant-induced_skin_necrosis"

Anticonvulsant hypersensitivity syndrome

Anticonvulsant hypersensitivity syndrome can be seen with diphenylhydantoin, phenobarbital, carbamazepine, lamotrigine, and other anticonvulsants, characterized by a skin eruption that is initially morbilliform. As this syndrome can present secondary to multiple anticonvulsants, the general term "anticonvulsant hypersensitivity syndrome" is favored over the original descriptive term "dilantin hypersensitivity syndrome."
Source (edited): "http://en.wikipedia.org/wiki/Anticonvulsant_hypersensitivity_syndrome"

Aquadynia

Aquadynia is a variant of aquagenic pruritus, and characterized by a widespread burning pain that lasts 15 to 45 minutes after water exposure.
Source (edited): "http://en.wikipedia.org/wiki/Aquadynia"

Aquagenic keratoderma

Aquagenic keratoderma, also known as **acquired aquagenic palmoplantar keratoderma**, **transient reactive papulotranslucent acrokeratoderma**, **aquagenic syringeal acrokeratoderma**, and **aquagenic wrinkling of the palms**, is a skin condition characterized by the development of white papules on the palms after water exposure.

An association with cystic fibrosis has been suggested.
Source (edited): "http://en.wikipedia.org/wiki/Aquagenic_keratoderma"

Arterial insufficiency ulcer

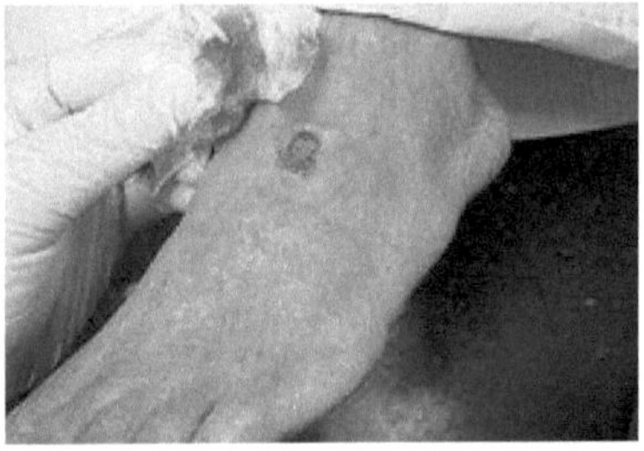

A 71-year-old diabetic male smoker with severe peripheral arterial disease presented with a dorsal foot ulceration (2.5 cm X 2.4cm) that had been chronically open for nearly 2 years.

Arterial insufficiency ulcers (also known as "Ischemic ulcers") are mostly localed on the lateral surface of the ankle or the distal digits.

Etiology

The ulcers are caused by lack of blood flow to the capillary beds of the lower extremities. When pressure is placed on the skin, the skin is damaged and is unable to be repaired due to the lack of blood perfusing the tissue. The wound has a characteristic deep, punched out look, often extending down to the tendons. The wounds are very painful.
Source (edited): "http://en.wikipedia.org/wiki/Arterial_insufficiency_ulcer"

Arteriosclerosis obliterans

Arteriosclerosis obliterans is an occlusive arterial disease most prominently affecting the abdominal aorta and the small- and medium-sized arteries of the lower extremities, which may lead to absent dorsalis pedis, posterior tibial, and/or popliteal artery pulses.
Source (edited): "http://en.wikipedia.org/wiki/Arteriosclerosis_obliterans"

Atrophic lichen planus

Atrophic lichen planus is a rare variant of lichen planus, and characterized by the presence of a few well-demarcated, white-bluish papules or plaques with central superficial atrophy.

Orally: The typical appearances of the atrophic (erosive) form of lichen planus are the keratotic white areas associated with erythema and shallow ulcerations. The lesions are usually less extensive and more prominent on the posterior buccal mucosa(Edward W. Odell).

Source (edited): "http://en.wikipedia.org/wiki/Atrophic_lichen_planus"

Atrophoderma of Pasini and Pierini

Atrophoderma of Pasini and Pierini (also known as "Dyschromic and atrophic variation of scleroderma," "Morphea plana atrophica," "Sclérodermie atrophique d'emblée") is a disease characterized by large lesions with a sharp peripheral border dropping into a depression with no outpouching, which, on biopsy, elastin is normal, while collagen may be thickened. Atrophoderma of Pasini and Pierini affects less than 200,000 Americans and is classified as a rare disease by http://rarediseases.info.nih.gov...") The disease results in round or oval patches of hyper-pigmented skin. The darkened skin patches may sometimes have a bluish or purplish hue when they first appear and are often smooth to the touch and hairless.

Source (edited): "http://en.wikipedia.org/wiki/Atrophoderma_of_Pasini_and_Pierini"

Atypical chronic pain syndrome

Atypical chronic pain syndrome is characterized by patients who will present to dermatologists with complaints of burning, pain, or dysesthesias in the skin or mucous membranes for which no identifiable pathology can be found.

Source (edited): "http://en.wikipedia.org/wiki/Atypical_chronic_pain_syndrome"

Atypical lichen myxedematosus

Atypical lichen myxedematosus (also known as "Intermediate lichen myxedematosus") is a skin condition caused by fibroblasts producing abnormally large amounts of mucopolysaccharides.

Source (edited): "http://en.wikipedia.org/wiki/Atypical_lichen_myxedematosus"

Atypical tuberous myxedema

Atypical tuberous myxedema, also known as Jadassohn–Dosseker syndrome, is thought to represent a pure nodular variant of lichen myxedematosus.

Source (edited): "http://en.wikipedia.org/wiki/Atypical_tuberous_myxedema"

Autoimmune estrogen dermatitis

Autoimmune estrogen dermatitis presents as a cyclic skin disorder that may appear eczematous, papular, bullous, or urticarial. with pruritus typically present, skin eruptions that may be chronic but which are exacerbated premenstrually or occur immediately following menses.

Source (edited): "http://en.wikipedia.org/wiki/Autoimmune_estrogen_dermatitis"

Autoimmune progesterone dermatitis

Autoimmune progesterone dermatitis may appear as urticarial papules, deep gyrate lesions, papulovesicular lesions, an eczematous eruption, or as targetoid lesions. Autoimmune progesterone dermatitis initially manifests with eye symptoms, e.g. burning, and progresses into rashes. Its relapsing-remitting pattern in women correspond to the progesterone levels durning the menstrual cycle, which spike twice a month. It is an extremely rare disease, only perhaps 50 cases have ever been reported.

Source (edited): "http://en.wikipedia.org/wiki/Autoimmune_progesterone

_dermatitis"

Autosensitization dermatitis

Autosensitization dermatitis (or **cutaneous autosensitization**) presents with the development of widespread dermatitis or dermatitis distant from a local inflammatory focus, a process referred to as autoeczematization.

Source (edited): "http://en.wikipedia.org/wiki/Autosensitization_dermatitis"

B-mannosidase deficiency

B-mannosidase deficiency is a rare autosomal recessive condition characterized by angiokeratomas similar to those seen with Fabry disease.

Source (edited): "http://en.wikipedia.org/wiki/B-mannosidase_deficiency"

Balloon cell nevus

Balloon cell nevi are a cutaneous condition characterized histologically by large, pale, polyhedral balloon cells.
Source (edited): "http://en.wikipedia.org/wiki/Balloon_cell_nevus"

Benign cephalic histiocytosis

Benign cephalic histiocytosis (also known as "Histiocytosis with intracytoplasmic worm-like bodies") is a rare cutaneous condition affecting boys and girls equally, characterized by skin lesions that initially present on the head in all cases, often the cheeks, eyelids, forehead, and ears.

Source (edited): "http://en.wikipedia.org/wiki/Benign_cephalic_histiocytosis"

Benign symmetric lipomatosis

Benign symmetric lipomatosis (also known as **Benign symmetric lipomatosis of Launois–Bensaude** and **Madelung's disease**) is a cutaneous condition characterized by extensive symmetric fat deposits in the head, neck, and shoulder girdle area. Named after German surgeon Otto Wilhelm Madelung who was the first to give a detailed description of it, the condition is very rare with an estimated incidence rate of 1 in 25,000 and affecting males up to 30 times more frequently than females. The etiology of the disease remains unknown, but there is a strong correlation with alcohol abuse. Traditionally the treatment is mainly surgical consisting of the removal of the lipomas, although recent study has proposed Phosphatidylcholine injection as a possible alternative.

Source (edited): "http://en.wikipedia.org/wiki/Benign_symmetric_lipomatosis"

Beryllium granuloma

Beryllium granulomas is a skin condition caused by granulomatous inflammation of the skin which may follow accident laceration, usually in the occupational setting.
Source (edited): "http://en.wikipedia.org/wiki/Beryllium_granuloma"

Bier spots

Bier spots are small, light macules usually found on the arms and legs of young adults, in which the intervening skin may seem erthematous but blanches with pressure so that these light macules disappear. This is a benign physiologic vascular anomaly of no significance clinically.

Source (edited): "http://en.wikipedia.org/wiki/Bier_spots"

Biliary pruritus

Biliary pruritus is caused by chronic liver disease with obstructive jaundice, characterized by a severe generalized itchy sensation.

Source (edited): "http://en.wikipedia.org/wiki/Biliary_pruritus"

Black heel and palm

Black heel and palm (also known as "Calcaneal petechiae," "Chromidrose plantaire," "Post-traumatic punctate intraepidermal hemorrhage," "Tache noir," and "Talon noir") is a skin condition characterized by a sudden shower of minute, black, punctate macules occurring most often on the posterior edge of the plantar surface of one or both heels.

Source (edited): "http://en.wikipedia.org/wiki/Black_heel_and_palm"

Blackhead

A **blackhead** (medically known as an **open comedo**, plural **comedones**) is a yellow or blackish bump or plug on the skin. A blackhead is a type of acne vulgaris. Contrary to the common belief that it is caused by poor hygiene, blackheads are caused by excess oils that have accumulated in the sebaceous gland's duct. The substance found in these bumps mostly consists of keratin and modified sebum (an oily secretion of the sebaceous gland), which darkens as it oxidizes. Clogged hair follicles, where blackheads often occur, reflect light irregularly to produce a blackhead's "black" hue. For this reason, the blockage might not necessarily look black when extracted from the pore, but may have a more yellow-brown colour as a result of its melanin content.

In contrast, a "whitehead" (more commonly known as a pimple or a closed comedo) is a follicle that is filled with the same material, sebum, but lacks a microscopic opening to the skin surface. Since the air cannot reach the follicle, the material is not oxidized, and remains white.

Source (edited): "http://en.wikipedia.org/wiki/Blackhead"

Blastic NK-cell lymphoma

Blastic NK-cell lymphoma is a cutaneous condition characterized by multiple, rapidly expanding plaques.

Source (edited): "http://en.wikipedia.org/wiki/Blastic_NK-cell_lymphoma"

Blau syndrome

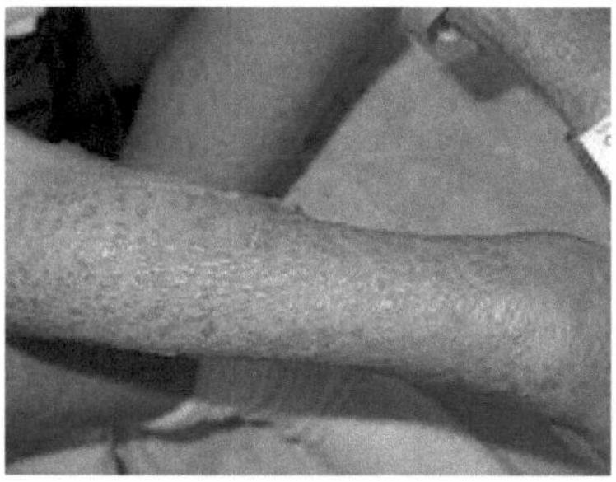

Multiple, reddish-brown papules coalescing over the right arm in a boy with Blau syndrome

Blau syndrome is characterized by familial granulomatous arthritis, iritis, and skin granulomas, comprising an autosomal dominantly inherited syndrome that overlaps both sarcoidosis and granuloma annulare. Restated, Blau syndrome is a rare autosomal dominant disorder characterized by granulomatous polyarthritis, panuveitis, cranial neuropathies, and exanthema. Camptodactyly is another feature, and Crohn's disease occurs in 30%.

It is associated with mutations in the *NOD2* gene.

Source (edited): "http://en.wikipedia.org/wiki/Blau_syndrome"

Blepharophyma

Blepharophyma refers to chronic swelling of eyelids, mainly due to sebaceous gland hyperplasia.

Source (edited): "http://en.wikipedia.org/wiki/Blepharophyma"

Blue nevus

Blue nevus (also known as "Blue neuronevus," "Dermal melanocytoma," and "Nevus bleu") is a type of melanocytic nevus.

It is usually described as non-cancerous, but can be malignant.

Types

Blue nevi may be divided into the following types:

- Blue nevus of Jadassohn-Tiche
- Cellular blue nevus
- Epithelioid blue nevus
- Deep penetrating nevus
- Amelanotic blue nevus
- Malignant blue nevus

Source (edited): "http://en.wikipedia.org/wiki/Blue_nevus"

Blue nevus of Jadassohn–Tièche

Blue nevus of Jadassohn–Tièche (also known as a "Common blue nevus," and "Nevus ceruleus") is a cutaneous condition characterized by a steel-blue papule or nodule.

Source (edited): "http://en.wikipedia.org/wiki/Blue_nevus_of_Jadassohn%E2%80%93Ti%C3%A8che"

Bonnet–Dechaume–Blanc syndrome

Bonnet–Dechaume–Blanc syndrome (also known as "Wyburn–Mason syndrome") is a rare condition characterized by a vascular malformation extending from the craniofacial to the orbital regions and brain.

It was characterized in 1938. The term "Wyburn–Mason syndrome" derives from a characterization made in 1943.

It is sometimes considered a phakomatosis.

Source (edited): "http://en.wikipedia.org/wiki/Bonnet%E2%80%93Dechaume%E2%80%93Blanc_syndrome"

Brachioradial pruritus

Brachioradial pruritus is becoming increasingly common, presenting in patients who are usually fair skinned, affluent, and middle aged that indulge in golf, tennis, sailing, or other leisure outdoor activities in sunny climates.

Treatment with lamotrigine has been reported.

Source (edited): "http://en.wikipedia.org/wiki/Brachioradial_pruritus"

Breast eczema

Breast eczema (also known as "Nipple eczema") may affect the nipples, areolae, or surrounding skin, with eczema of the nipples being of the moist type with oozing and crusting, in which painful fissuring is frequently seen, especially in nursing mothers.

Source (edited): "http://en.wikipedia.org/wiki/Breast_eczema"

Bromidrosiphobia

Bromidrosiphobia is a neurosis in which a person is convinced that his/her sweat has a repugnant odor that keeps other people away. The patient is unable to accept any evidence to the contrary. Three-quarters of patients with bromidrosiphobia are male, with an average age of 25. Pimozide may be beneficial. It may be an early symptom of schizophrenia.

Source (edited): "http://en.wikipedia.org/wiki/Bromidrosiphobia"

Bromoderma

Bromoderma, also known as **bromoderma tuberosum**, is a dermatological condition characterized by an eruption of papules and pustules on the skin. It is caused by hypersensitivity to bromides, such as those found in certain drugs. There is at least one reported case of bromoderma caused by excessive consumption of a soft drink containing brominated vegetable oil.

Source (edited): "http://en.wikipedia.org/wiki/Bromoderma"

Bullous drug reaction

Bullous drug reaction (also known as a "Bullous drug eruption," "Generalized bullous fixed drug eruption," and "Multilocular bullous fixed drug eruption") most commonly refers to a drug reaction in the erythema multiforme group. These are uncommon reactions to medications, with an incidence of 0.4 to 1..2 per million person-years for toxic epidermal necrolysis and 1.2 to 6.0 per million person-years for Stevens-Johnson syndrome. The primary skin lesions are large erythemas (faintly discernable even after confluence), most often irregularly distributed and of a characteristic purplish-livid color, at times with flaccid blisters.
Source (edited): "http://en.wikipedia.org/wiki/Bullous_drug_reaction"

Bullous lichen planus

Bullous lichen planus (also known as "Vesiculobullous lichen planus") is a rare variant of lichen planus, characterized by the development of vesicles and bullae with the skin lesions.
Source (edited): "http://en.wikipedia.org/wiki/Bullous_lichen_planus"

Bullous lymphedema

Bullous lymphedema is a skin condition that usually occurs with poorly controlled edema related to heart failure and fluid overload, and compression results in healing.
Source (edited): "http://en.wikipedia.org/wiki/Bullous_lymphedema"

Bullous pemphigoid

Bullous pemphigoid, also referred to as **BP**, is an acute or chronic autoimmune skin disease, involving the formation of blisters, more appropriately known as bullae, at the space between the skin layers epidermis and dermis.

Pathophysiology

The bullae are formed by an immune reaction, initiated by the formation of IgG autoantibodies targeting the type XVII collagen component of hemidesmosomes. It can also rarely involve the mucous membranes. Following antibody targeting, a cascade of immunomodulators results in a variable surge of neutrophils, lymphocytes and eosinophils coming to the affected area. Unclear events subsequently result in a separation along the dermal-epidermal junction and eventually stretch bullae.

Presentation

Clinically the earliest lesions may appear urticarial (like hives). Tense bullae eventually erupt, most commonly at the inner thighs and upper arms but the trunk and extremities are frequently both involved. Any part of the skin surface can be involved. Milia are more common with epidermolysis bullosa acquisita (EBA), because of the deeper antigenic targets. A more ring-like configuration, with a central depression or centrally collapsed bullae may indicate linear IgA disease. The disease may be acute, but typically will wax and wane.

Diagnosis

Diagnosis is based on two biopsies of the skin, one submitted for routine H &E staining and one for immunofluorescence studies.

Treatment

Treatments include Class I topical steroids (clobetasol, halobetasol, etc.) which in some studies have proven to be equally as effective as systemic, or pill, therapy and somewhat safer. However, in difficult to manage or widespread cases, systemic prednisone and powerful steroid-free immunosuppressant medications such as methotrexate, azathioprine or mycophenolate mofetil may be appropriate.

Epidemiology

Many mammals can be afflicted, including dogs, cats, pigs, and horses, as well as humans. Very rarely seen in children, it usually occurs in people 70 years of age and older. It is very rare in dogs; on average, three cases are diagnosed around the world each year.

At least one study indicates the incidence might be increasing in the United Kingdom.
Source (edited): "http://en.wikipedia.org/wiki/Bullous_pemphigoid"

CD30+ cutaneous T-cell lymphoma

CD30+ cutaneous T-cell lymphoma (also known as "Primary cutaneous anaplastic large cell lymphoma") is a cutaneous condition characterized by solitary of localized skin lesions that have a tendency to ulcerate.

Source (edited): "http://en.wikipedia.org/wiki/CD30%2B_cutaneous_T-cell_lymphoma"

CREST syndrome

The **limited cutaneous** form of **systemic scleroderma** (lcSSc) is often referred to as **CREST syndrome**. "CREST" is an acronym for the five main features:

- Calcinosis
- Raynaud's syndrome
- Esophageal dysmotility
- Sclerodactyly
- Telangiectasia

It is a form of systemic scleroderma associated with antibodies against centromeres and usually spares the kidneys. If the lungs are involved it is usually in the form of pulmonary arterial hypertension.

CREST is a systemic inflammatory rheumatic disease and usually results in more pathologies than the five symptoms above.

Patients with lcSSc commonly and slowly produce a pulmonary artery hypertension which can result in heart failure. Blood vessel thrombosis and arteriosclerosis has also led to the necessity of amputation of fingers. Open leg sores can result from burst blood vessels and thin skin, leading to chronic infections. Other symptoms of CREST patients can be exhaustion, weakness, difficulties with breathing, dizziness and badly healing wounds.

The origin of CREST lies in the immune system. There is production of anti-nuclear and anti-centromere antibodies, although it is not known if these antibodies are involved in the cause of the symptoms of the disease. There is no known infectious cause.

There is no cure for this disease as there is no cure for scleroderma in general. It slowly progresses and should be examined and treated as soon as it has been diagnosed with immunosuppressives and other medications. There are treatments that can ameliorate the symptoms of esophageal reflux, pulmonary hypertension and Raynaud phenomonon.

Source (edited): "http://en.wikipedia.org/wiki/CREST_syndrome"

Calcinosis cutis

Calcinosis cutis (or **cutaneous calcification**) is a type of calcinosis wherein calcium deposits form in the skin. A variety of factors can result in this condition. The most common source is dystrophic calcification, which occurs in soft tissue as a response to injury. In dogs, calcinosis cutis is virtually pathognomonic for Canine Cushing's syndrome.

Types

Calcinosis cutis may be divided into the following types:

- Dystrophic calcinosis cutis
- Metastatic calcinosis cutis
- Iatrogenic calcinosis cutis
- Traumatic calcinosis cutis
- Idiopathic scrotal calcinosis
- Subepidermal calcified nodule
- Tumoral calcinosis
- Osteoma cutis

Causes

Calcinosis may be the results of a variety of causes such as:

- Trauma to the region
- Inflammation (bug bites, acne)
- Varicose veins
- Infections
- Tumors (malignant or benign)
- Diseases of connective tissue
- Hypercalcemia
- Hyperphosphatemia

Gallery

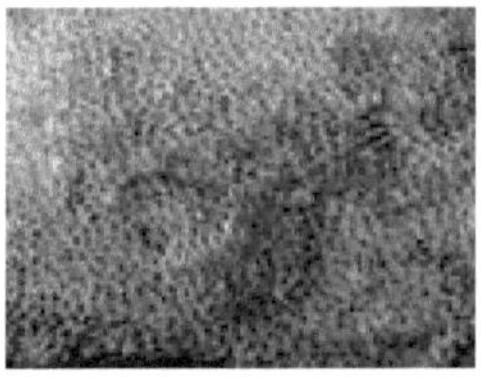

Calcinosis cutis in a dog with Cushing's syndrome

Source (edited): "http://en.wikipedia.org/wiki/Calcinosis_cutis"

Camisa disease

Camisa disease (or **Vohwinkel variant with ichthyosis**) is the variant form of Vohwinkel syndrome, characterized by ichthyosis and normal hearing.

It is associated with loricrin.

It was characterized in 1984 and 1988.

Source (edited): "http://en.wikipedia.org/wiki/Camisa_disease"

Carbon stain

Carbon stains are a skin condition characterized by a discoloration of the skin from embedded carbon, usually occurring in children from careless use of firearms or firecrackers, or from puncture wound by a pencil, which may leave a permanent black mark of embedded graphite, easily mistaken for metastatic melanoma.

Source (edited): "http://en.wikipedia.org/wiki/Carbon_stain"

Caviar tongue

Caviar tongue is a condition characterized by purplish venous ectasias commonly found on the undersurface of the tongue after the age of fifty.

Source (edited): "http://en.wikipedia.org/wiki/Caviar_tongue"

Cellular blue nevus

Cellular blue nevi are a cutaneous condition characterized by large, firm, blue or blue-black nodules.

Source (edited): "http://en.wikipedia.org/wiki/Cellular_blue_nevus"

Centrifugal abdominal lipodystrophy

Centrifugal abdominal lipodystrophy (also known as "Centrifugal lipodystrophy," "Lipodystrophia centrifugalis abdominalis infantalis") is a skin condition characterized by areas of subcutaneous fat loss that slowly enlarge.

Source (edited): "http://en.wikipedia.org/wiki/Centrifugal_abdominal_lipodystrophy"

Centrofacial lentiginosis

Centrofacial lentiginosis is a cutaneous condition characterized by lentigines on the nose and adjacent cheeks.

Source (edited): "http://en.wikipedia.org/wiki/Centrofacial_lentiginosis"

Cheilitis

Cheilitis is a medical condition involving inflammation of the lip.

It is associated with many conditions, including megaloblastic anemia from vitamin B deficiency, iron deficiency anemia (which in severe cases can lead to Plummer-Vinson syndrome) and oral candidiasis. It can also be a symptom of allergies, such as allergy to Balsam of Peru. Cheilitis can also be caused by taking the (retinoid) drug Isotretinoin (brand name Roaccutane) (BNF84).

It may also be a pre-malignant lesion for squamous cell carcinoma.

Types

Cheilitis may be divided into the following types:

- Cheilitis exfoliativa
- Allergic contact cheilitis
- Actinic cheilitis
- Cheilitis glandularis
- Angular cheilitis (Perlèche)
- Plasma cell cheilitis

Source (edited): "http://en.wikipedia.org/wiki/Cheilitis"

Cheilitis exfoliativa

Cheilitis exfoliativa is an inflammatory condition of the lips, in which they may be covered with crusts.

Source (edited): "http://en.wikipedia.org/wiki/Cheilitis_exfoliativa"

Cheilitis glandularis

Cheilitis glandularis is a conditions characterized by swelling and eversion of the lower lip. Cheilitis glandularis is an acquired disorder, of unknown aetiology, characterized by swelling, ulceration, crusting, mucous gland hyperplasia, abscesses, and sinus tracts.

Source (edited): "http://en.wikipedia.org/wiki/Cheilitis_glandularis"

Cheilitis granulomatosa

Cheilitis granulomatosa (also known as "Granulomatous cheilitis," and "Orofacial granulomatosis") is a condition characterized by a sudden onset and progressive course terminating in chronic enlargement of the lips.

Source (edited): "http://en.wikipedia. org/wiki/Cheilitis_granulomatosa"

Chemical burn

A **chemical burn** occurs when living tissue is exposed to a corrosive substance such as a strong acid or base. Chemical burns follow standard burn classification and may cause extensive tissue damage. The main types of irritant and/or corrosive products are: acids, bases, oxidizers, solvents, reducing agents and alkylants. Additionally, chemical burns can be caused by some types of chemical weapons e.g. vesicants such as mustard gas and Lewisite, or urticants such as phosgene oxime.

Chemical burns may:

- need no source of heat,
- occur immediately on contact,
- be extremely painful, or
- not be immediately evident or noticeable

Presentation

The exact symptoms of a chemical burn depend on the chemical involved. Symptoms include itching, bleaching or darkening of skin, burning sensations, trouble breathing, coughing blood and/or tissue necrosis. Common sources of chemical burns include sulfuric acid (HSO), hydrochloric acid (HCl), lye (NaOH), lime (CaO), and silver nitrate (AgNO). Chemical burns may occur through direct contact on body surfaces including skin and eyes, inhalation, and ingestion. Lipophilic substances that diffuse efficiently in human tissue, e.g. hydrofluoric acid, sulfur mustard and dimethyl sulfate, may not react immediately, but produce the burns and inflammation hours after the contact. Chemical fabrication, mining, medicine, and related professional fields are examples of occupations where chemical burns may occur.

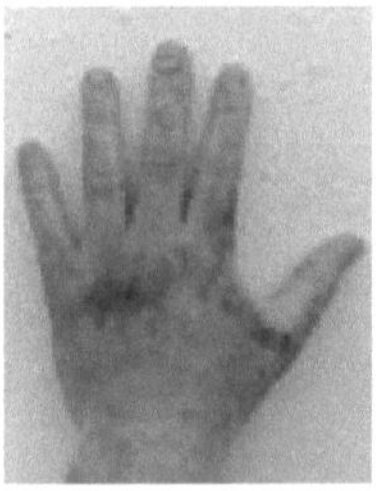

Chemical burn caused by exposure to a sodium hydroxide solution.

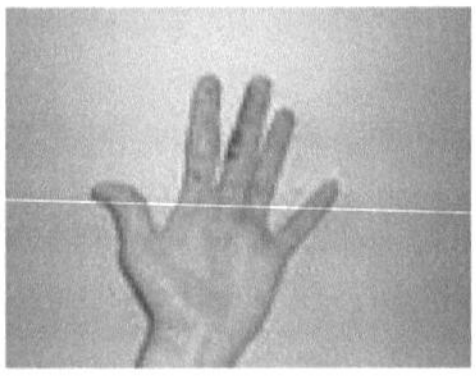

Second degree chemical burn, resulting from prolonged contact with concentrated AgNO, on the left hand of a caucasian woman.

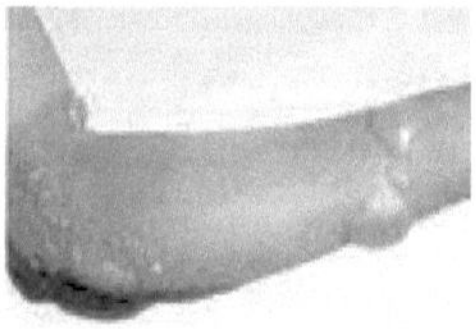

Chemical burns to the arm, caused by a blister agent e.g. mustard gas.

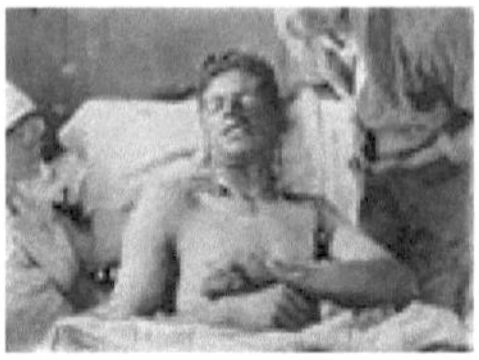

Chemical burns caused by exposure to mustard gas during the First World War.

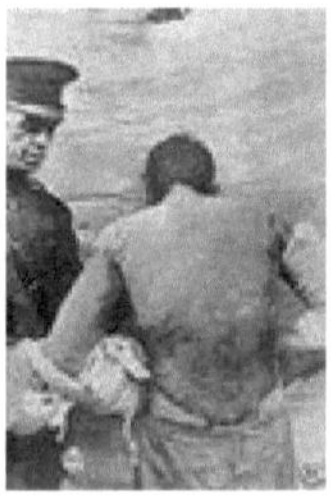

Soldier with severe mustard gas burns to back and arms circa 1918. These burns are severe enough to be life-threatening.

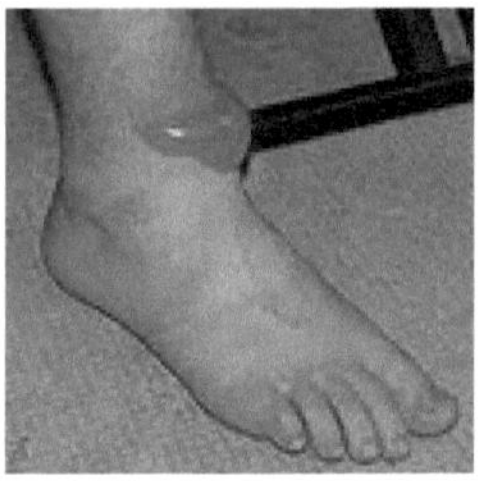

Severe skin burns with roundup are very rare, but possible

Source (edited): "http://en.wikipedia. org/wiki/Chemical_burn"

Chemotherapy-induced hyperpigmentation

Chemotherapy-induced hyperpigmentation is caused by many chemotherapeutic agents (especially the antibiotics bleomycin, and daunorubicin) and the alkylating agents (cyclophosphamide and busulfan).

Source (edited): "http://en.wikipedia. org/wiki/Chemotherapy-induced_hyperpigmentation"

Chilblain lupus erythematosus

Chilblain lupus erythematosus (also known as "Chilblain lupus erythematosus of Hutchinson") is a chronic, unremitting form of lupus erythematosus with the fingertips, rims of ears, calves, and heels affected, especially in women.

Source (edited): "http://en.wikipedia. org/wiki/Chilblain_lupus_erythematosus"

Childhood dermatomyositis

Childhood dermatomyositis is a connective-tissue disease related to polymyositis, characterized by inflammation of the muscles and the skin. It differs from adult dermatomyositis in several ways, and has two common variants. The more common form is the "Brunsting type," in which slow, progressive muscle weakness with calcinosis can be easily treated with corticosteroids. The second type is known as "Banker type," characterized by a vasculitis of the muscles and gastrointestinal tract, rapid onset of severe weakness, steroid unresponsiveness, and high death date.

Pathology

Dermatomyositis is confirmed by proximal muscle weakness, an electromyography with a characteristic "spike and wave" pattern, and abnormal CPK or aldolase levels. Conclusive diagnosis requires a muscle biopsy that shows perifascicular infiltration of inflammatory cells.

Treatment

The more common type of dermatomyositis, the unicyclic "Brunsting type", responds well to corticosteroids and typically disappears within six months of treatment. Muscular calcifications can be surgically removed, but doing so may result in poor wound healing; calcifications can be reduced with bisphosphonates.

Children with the rare polycyclic form of dermatomyositis can also be treated with corticosteroids and methotrexate, but respond poorly. Muscle cells that die during the inflammatory phase of dermatomyositis are nonrenewable, which can lead to permanent weakness.

Source (edited): "http://en.wikipedia.org/wiki/Childhood_dermatomyositis"

Childhood linear IgA disease

Childhood linear IgA disease (also known as "Chronic bullous disease of childhood") is an acquired, self-limited bullous disease that may begin by the time the patient is age 2 to 3 and usually remits by age 13.

Source (edited): "http://en.wikipedia.org/wiki/Childhood_linear_IgA_disease"

Childhood systemic lupus erythematosus

Childhood systemic lupus erythematosus generally presents between the ages of 3 and 15, with girls outnumbering boys 4:1, and typical skin manifestations being butterfly eruption on the face and photosensitivity.

Source (edited): "http://en.wikipedia.org/wiki/Childhood_systemic_lupus_erythematosus"

Chronic actinic dermatitis

Chronic actinic dermatitis (also known as "Actinic reticuloid," "Chronic photosensitivity dermatitis," "Persistent light reactivity," and "Photosensitive eczema") is a condition where a subject's skin becomes inflamed due to a reaction to sunlight or artificial light. CAD patients often suffer from other related conditions of the skin that results in dermatitis in response to a variety of stimulus (e.g., flowers, sunscreens, cosmetics, etc.).

Source (edited): "http://en.wikipedia.org/wiki/Chronic_actinic_dermatitis"

Chronic erythema nodosum

Chronic erythema nodosum (also known as "Erythema nodosum migrans," "Subacute migratory panniculitis of Vilanova and Piñol", and "Subacute nodular migratory panniculitis") is a form of septal panniculitis that is much less common than acute erythema nodosum.

Source (edited): "http://en.wikipedia.org/wiki/Chronic_erythema_nodosum"

Chronic radiodermatitis

Chronic radiodermatitis occurs with chronic exposure to "sub-erythema" doses of ionizing radiation over a pro-

longed period, producing varying degrees of damage to the skin and its underlying parts after a variable latent period of several months to several decades. In the past this type of radiation reaction occurred most frequently in radiologists and radiation technicians who were constantly exposed to ionizing radiation. Restated, chronic radiodermatitis, squamous and basal cell carcinomas may develop months to years after radiation exposure. Clinically, chronic radiodermatitis presents as atrophic indurated plaques, often whitish or yellowish, with telangiectasia, sometimes with hyperkeratosis.
Source (edited): "http://en.wikipedia.org/wiki/Chronic_radiodermatitis"

Chronic urticaria

Chronic urticaria (also known as "Ordinary urticaria") is defined as the presence of evanescent wheals which persist for greater than six weeks.
Source (edited): "http://en.wikipedia.org/wiki/Chronic_urticaria"

Chronic vesiculobullous hand eczema

Chronic vesiculobullous hand eczema presents with lesions that may be hyperkeratotic, scaling, and fissures, and the "dyshidrosiform" pattern may be recognized only during exacerbations. Females outnumber names by 3:1, and there is a tendency for the pruritic 1- to 2-mm vesicles to be most pronounced at the sides of the fingers.
Source (edited): "http://en.wikipedia.org/wiki/Chronic_vesiculobullous_hand_eczema"

Cicatricial pemphigoid

Cicatricial pemphigoid (also known as "Benign mucosal pemphigoid," "Benign mucous membrane pemphigoid," "Ocular pemphigus," and "Scarring pemphigoid") is a rare chronic autoimmune subepithelial blistering disease characterized by erosive skin lesions of the mucous membranes and skin that results in scarring of at least some sites of involvement.

Cicatricial pemphigoid has been referred to by a variety of designations based largely on its site of involvements, with examples of such terminology including "desquamative gingivitis," "ocular pemphigus," and "benign mucous membrane pemphigoid." However, currently "...such designations are thought to be confusing or somewhat misleadings (e.g., pemphigus in this context is a misnomer , and this disorder is hardly benign given the extend of morbidity it can cause)."

Presentation

In mucous membrane pemphigoid, the autoimmune reaction occurs in the skin, specifically at the level of the basement membrane, which connects the lower skin layer (dermis) to the upper skin layer (epidermis) and keeps it attached to the body.

When the condition is active, the basement membrane is dissolved by the antibodies produced, and areas of skin lift away at the base, causing hard blisters which scar if they burst. In other words, this is a desquamating/blistering disease in which the epithelium "unzips" from the underlying connective tissue, allowing fluid to gather that subsequently manifest as bullae, or blisters.

The autoimmune reaction most commonly affects the mouth, causing lesions in the gingiva or gums, but it can also affect areas of mucous membrane elsewhere in the body, such as the sinuses, genitals and anus. When the cornea of the eye is affected, repeated scarring may result in blindness.

Nikolsky's sign (gentle lateral pressure on unaffected mucosa or skin raises a bulla. If no lesions are present on examination it may be useful way of demonstrating reduced epithelial adhesion. In (Pemphigus) the epithelium tends to disintegrate rather than form a bulla. Edward W. Odell.

Diagnosis

Diagnostic techniques:

- antibodies (IgG) precipitates complement (C3) in the lamina lucida of the basement membrane.
- Circulating auto-antibodies to BP-1 antigen (located in hemidesmosome). 50% have BP-2.
- Positive Nikolsky sign.
- IgG, C3 deposition at BM creating smooth line in immunofluorescent analysis.

Source (edited): "http://en.wikipedia.org/wiki/Cicatricial_pemphigoid"

Circumostomy eczema

Circumostomy eczema frequently occurs after an ileostomy or colostomy in which there is eczematization or autosensitization of the surrounding skin.
Source (edited): "http://en.wikipedia.org/wiki/Circumostomy_eczema"

Cold panniculitis

Cold panniculitis is a skin condition characterized by inflammation of the subcutaneous fat after exposure to cold, most often seen in infants and young children. This condition has been described in children who suck ice or popsicles, and therefore is sometimes referred to as "popsicle panniculitis."

Source (edited): "http://en.wikipedia.org/wiki/Cold_panniculitis"

Colloid milium

Colloid milium is a skin condition characterized by a translucent, flesh-colored, or slightly yellow 1- to 5-mm papule.

Treatment

There is no entirely successful treatment for colloid milium. Attempted treatments with varying results include:

- cryotherapy
- Er:YAG laser
- dermabrasion
- diathermy
- systemic ascorbic acid
- exfoliating agents

Source (edited): "http://en.wikipedia.org/wiki/Colloid_milium"

Congenital generalized lipodystrophy

Congenital generalized lipodystrophy (also known as **Berardinelli–Seip syndrome**) is a rare autosomal dominant skin condition, characterized by an extreme paucity of fat in the subcutaneous tissues.

Presentation

Berardinelli-Seip congenital lipodystrophy is a rare autosomal recessive condition associating insulin resistance, absence of subcutaneous fat and muscular hypertrophy. With characteristic features like hepatomegaly, accelerated growth, muscle hypertrophy, lack of adipose tissue, hirsutism and hypertriglyceridemia. Common cardiovascular alterations related to this syndrome are cardiac hypertrophy and arterial hypertension. and it is associated with metabolic syndrome.

Source (edited): "http://en.wikipedia.org/wiki/Congenital_generalized_lipodystrophy"

Congenital hypertrophy of the lateral fold of the hallux

Congenital hypertrophy of the lateral fold of the hallux is a rare cutaneous condition of unknown pathology that present to newborns. The condition was "first described by Martinet et al. in 1984." This sometimes painful condition involves "an overgrowth of the soft tissue" that can partially cover the nail plate. The condition usually effects both extremities and the condition can later reverse spontaneously.

Source (edited): "http://en.wikipedia.org/wiki/Congenital_hypertrophy_of_the_lateral_fold_of_the_hallux"

Congenital self-healing reticulohistiocytosis

Congenital self-healing reticulohistiocytosis (also known as "Hashimoto–Pritzker disease," and "Hashimoto–Pritzker syndrome") is a condition that is a self-limited form of Langerhans cell histiocytosis.

Source (edited): "http://en.wikipedia.org/wiki/Congenital_self-healing_reticulohistiocytosis"

Coral cut

Coral cuts are a severe type of skin injury that may occur from the cuts of coral skeletons.

Source (edited): "http://en.wikipedia.org/wiki/Coral_cut"

Corneodermatoosseous syndrome

Corneodermatosseous syndrome (also known as "CDO syndrome") is an autosomal dominant condition with on-

set in infancy, characterized by corneal dystrophy, photophobia, diffuse palmoplantar keratoderma, distal onycholysis, skeletal abnormalities, with brachydactyly, short stature, and medullary narrowing of digits.
Source (edited): "http://en.wikipedia.org/wiki/Corneodermatoosseous_syndrome"

Cross syndrome

Cross–McKusick–Breen syndrome (also known as "Cross syndrome," "Hypopigmentation and microphthalmia," and "Oculocerebral-hypopigmentation syndrome") is an extremely rare disorder characterized by white skin, blond hair with yellow-gray metallic sheen, small eyes with cloudy corneas, jerky nystagmus, gingival fibromatosis and severe mental and physical retardation.

It was characterized in 1967.
Source (edited): "http://en.wikipedia.org/wiki/Cross_syndrome"

Cryofibrinogenemic purpura

Cryofibrinogenemic purpura is a skin condition that manifests as painful purpura with slow healing ulcerations and edema of both feet during winter months.
Source (edited): "http://en.wikipedia.org/wiki/Cryofibrinogenemic_purpura"

Cryoglobulinemic purpura

Cryoglobulinemic purpura is a skin condition characterized by purpura and occurring most frequently in multiple myeloma and macroglobulinemia.
Source (edited): "http://en.wikipedia.org/wiki/Cryoglobulinemic_purpura"

Cryoglobulinemic vasculitis

Cryoglobulinemic vasculitis is a skin condition presenting in roughly 15% of people with a circulating cryoprecipitable protein.
Source (edited): "http://en.wikipedia.org/wiki/Cryoglobulinemic_vasculitis"

Cutaneous B-cell lymphoma

Cutaneous B-cell lymphomas constitute a group of diseases that occur less commonly than cutaneous T-cell lymphoma, and are characterized histologically by B-cells that appear similar to those normally found in germinal centers of lymph nodes. Conditions included in this group are:

- Diffuse large B-cell lymphoma
- Primary cutaneous follicular lymphoma
- Primary cutaneous marginal zone lymphoma
- Intravascular large B-cell lymphoma
- Plasmacytoma
- Plasmacytosis

Source (edited): "http://en.wikipedia.org/wiki/Cutaneous_B-cell_lymphoma"

Cutaneous focal mucinosis

Cutaneous focal mucinosis is a skin condition characterized by a solitary nodule or papule.
Source (edited): "http://en.wikipedia.org/wiki/Cutaneous_focal_mucinosis"

Cutaneous lymphoid hyperplasia

Cutaneous lymphoid hyperplasia (also known as "borrelial lymphocytoma," "Lymphadenosis benigna cutis," "Lymphocytoma cutis," "Pseudolymphoma," "Pseudolymphoma of Spiegler and Fendt," "Sarcoidosis of Spiegler and Fendt," "Spiegler–Fendt lymphoid hyperplasia," and "Spiegler–Fendt sarcoid") refers to a groups of benign cutaneous disorders characterized by collections of lymphocytes, macrophages, and dendritic cells in the skin.

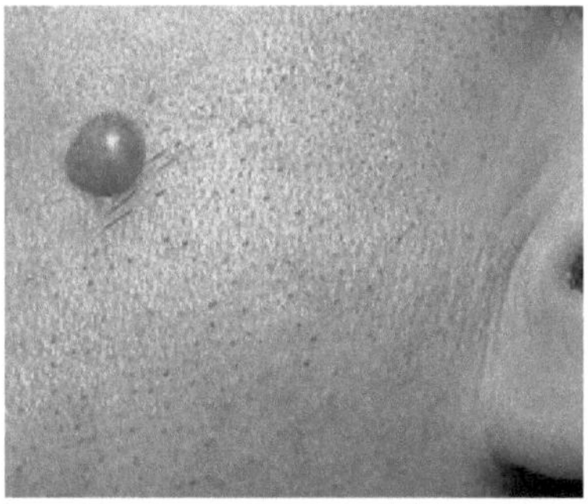
borrelial lymphocytoma on the cheek

Conditions included in this groups are:

- Cutaneous lymphoid hyperplasia with nodular pattern
- Cutaneous lymphoid hyperplasia with bandlike and perivascular patterns
- Jessner lymphocytic infiltrate of the skin

Source (edited): "http://en.wikipedia.org/wiki/Cutaneous_lymphoid_hyperplasia"

Cutaneous lymphoid hyperplasia with bandlike and perivascular patterns

Cutaneous lymphoid hyperplasia with bandlike and perivascular patterns is a condition of the skin characterized by skin lesions that clinically resemble mycosis fungoides.
Source (edited): "http://en.wikipedia.org/wiki/Cutaneous_lymphoid_hyperplasia_with_bandlike_and_perivascular_patterns"

Cutaneous lymphoid hyperplasia with nodular pattern

Cutaneous lymphoid hyperplasia with nodular pattern (also known as "Nodular pattern of cutaneous lymphoid hyperplasia") is a condition of the skin characterized by a solitary or localized cluster of asymptomatic erythematous to violaceous papules or nodules.
Source (edited): "http://en.wikipedia.org/wiki/Cutaneous_lymphoid_hyperplasia_with_nodular_pattern"

Cutaneous myelofibrosis

Cutaneous myelofibrosis is a rare skin condition characterized by dermal and subcutaneous nodules.
Source (edited): "http://en.wikipedia.org/wiki/Cutaneous_myelofibrosis"

Cutaneous sinus of dental origin

Cutaneous sinus of dental origin (also known as a "Dental sinus") is a condition in which a chronic periapical infection about a tooth produces a burrowing cordlike sinus tract that eventually appears beneath the surface of the gum, palate, or periorificial skin.
Source (edited): "http://en.wikipedia.org/wiki/Cutaneous_sinus_of_dental_origin"

Cutaneous small-vessel vasculitis

Cutaneous small-vessel vasculitis (also known as "Cutaneous leukocytoclastic angiitis," "Cutaneous leukocytoclastic vasculitis," "Cutaneous necrotizing venulitis," and "Hypersensitivity angiitis") is a inflammation of small blood vessels, characterized clinically by palpable purpura. Subtypes of small-vessel vasculitis include:

- Henoch-Schönlein purpura
- Acute hemorrhagic edema of infancy
- Urticarial vasculitis
- Cryoglobulinemic vasculitis
- Erythema elevatum diutinum
- Granuloma faciale

Leukocytoclastic vasculitis

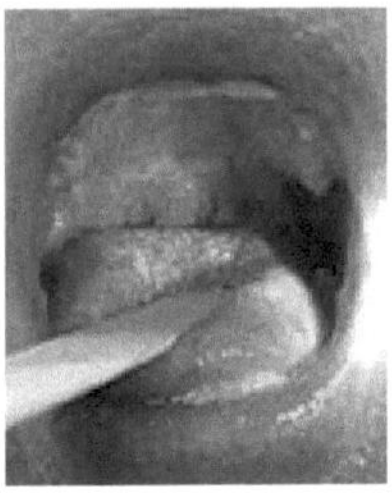

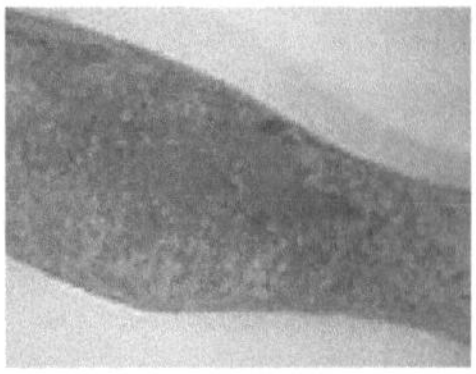

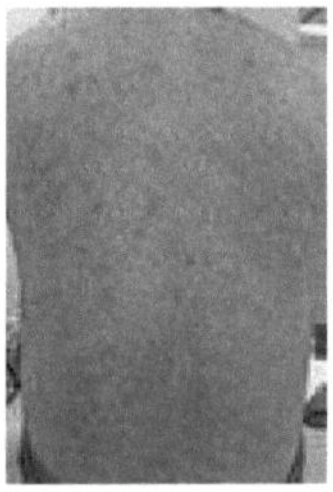

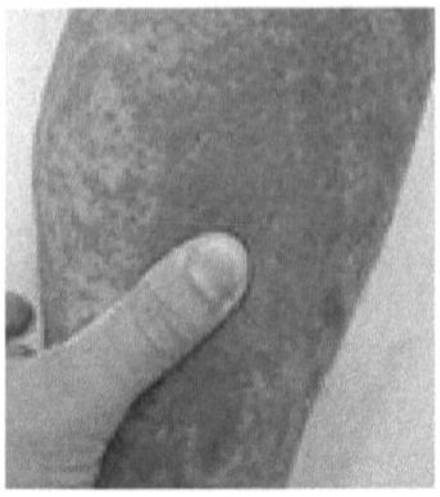

Source (edited): "http://en.wikipedia.org/wiki/Cutaneous_small-vessel_vasculitis"

Cytophagic histiocytic panniculitis

Cytophagic Histiocytic Panniculitis (CHP) was first described in 1980 by Winkelmann as a chronic histiocytic disease of the subcutaneous adipose tissue, which is characterized clinically by tender erythematous nodules, recurrent high fever, malaise, jaundice, organomegaly, serosal effusions, pancytopenia, hepatic dysfunction and Coagulation abnormalities. CHP may occur either isolated or as part of cutaneous manifestations of Hemophagocytic syndrome (HPS). CHP is a rare and often fatal form of panniculitis with multisystem involvement. But it can also present in a benign form involving only the subcutaneous tissue, thus having a broad clinical spectrum.
Source (edited): "http://en.wikipedia.org/wiki/Cytophagic_histiocytic_panniculitis"

Deep penetrating nevus

A **deep penetrating nevus** is a cutaneous condition characterized by cells with a smudged chromatin pattern.
Source (edited): "http://en.wikipedia.org/wiki/Deep_penetrating_nevus"

Defatting (medical)

Defatting is a medical term that describes the chemical dissolving of dermal lipids, from the skin, on contact with defatting agents. This can result in water loss from the affected area and cause the whitening and drying of the skin which can result in cracking, secondary infection and chemical irritant contact dermatitis.

Cause

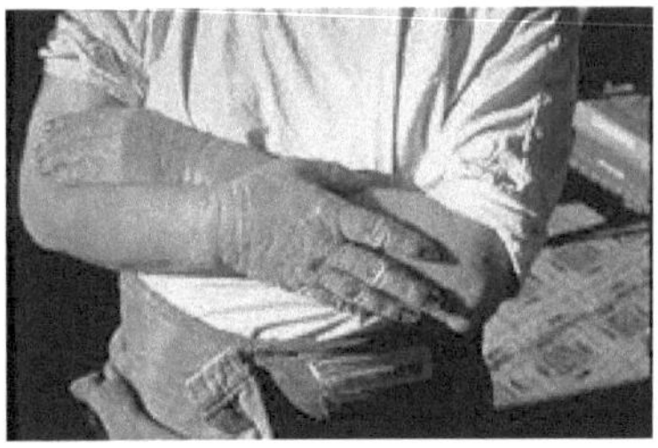

Prolonged defatting of the skin can lead to dermatitis. Here the hands and wrists of a worker display chronic dermatitis resulting from long term exposure to kerosene.

Defatting is caused from the exposure of human skin to a chemical substance, including alcohols, detergents, chemical solvents and motor oil. Aliphatic compounds (commonly found in kerosene) cause defatting action, with lower-boiling point aliphatics having the greatest defatting action and therefore the most potential to cause dermatitis. Aromatic solvents, such as Styrene also have a defatting capacity.

Prevention and care

Defatting can be prevented by wearing appropriate protective clothing such as gloves, lab coats and aprons when working with defatting agents on a regular basis.

Prolonged skin contact or chronic defatting of the skin increases the possibility of irritant contact dermatitis and has the potential to worsen pre-existing skin conditions. Patients with chronic dermatitis should be instructed to use non-irritating soaps and dishwashing liquids sparingly and to choose those with minimal defatting activity and a neutral pH.
Source (edited): "http://en.wikipedia.org/wiki/Defatting_(medical)"

Dermatitis repens

Dermatitis repens (also known as "Acrodermatitis continua," "Acrodermatitis perstans," "Pustular acrodermatitis," "Acrodermatitis continua of Hallopeau," "Acrodermatitis continua suppurativa Hallopeau," "Hallopeau's acrodermatitis,", "Hallopeau's acrodermatitis continua," and "Dermatitis repens Crocker") is a rare, sterile, pustular eruption of the fingers and toes that slowly extends proximally.
Source (edited): "http://en.wikipedia.org/wiki/Dermatitis_repens"

Dermatothlasia

Dermatothlasia is a cutaneous neurosis characterized by a person's uncontrollable desire to rub or pinch him/herself to form bruised areas on the skin, sometimes as a defense against pain elsewhere.
Source (edited): "http://en.wikipedia.org/wiki/Dermatothlasia"

Desmoplastic melanoma

Desmoplastic melanoma (also known as a "Neurotropic melanoma," or "Spindled melanoma") is a cutaneous condition characterized by a deeply infiltrating type of melanoma.
Source (edited): "http://en.wikipedia.org/wiki/Desmoplastic_melanoma"

Diabetic bulla

A **diabetic bulla** (also known as "Bullosis diabeticorum" and "Bullous eruption of diabetes mellitus") is a cutaneous condition characterized by a non-inflammatory, spontaneous, painless blister, often in acral locations (peripheral body parts, such as feet, toes, hands, fingers, ears or nose), seen in diabetic patients.
Source (edited): "http://en.wikipedia.org/wiki/Diabetic_bulla"

Diabetic cheiroarthropathy

Diabetic cheiroarthropathy is a cutaneous condition characterized by thickened skin and limited joint mobility of the hands and fingers, leading to flexion contractures, a condition associated with diabetes mellitus. and it is observed in roughly 30% of diabetic patients with longstanding disease.
Source (edited): "http://en.wikipedia.org/wiki/Diabetic_cheiroarthropathy"

Diabetic dermadrome

Diabetic dermadromes constitute a group of cutaneous conditions commonly seen in diabetic patients with longstanding disease. Conditions included in this group are:

- Acral dry gangrene
- Carotenosis
- Diabetic dermopathy
- Diabetic bulla
- Diabetic cheiroarthropathy
- Mal perforans
- Necrobiosis lipoidica
- **Limited joint mobility** is observed in roughly 30% of diabetic patients with longstanding disease.
- **Waxy skin** is observed in roughly 50%.

Source (edited): "http://en.wikipedia.org/wiki/Diabetic_dermadrome"

Diabetic dermopathy

Diabetic dermopathy (also known as "shin spots") is a type of skin lesion seen in people with diabetes mellitus. It is characterized by dull-red papules that progress to well-circumscribed, small, round, atrophic hyperpigmented skin lesions on the shins. It is the most common of several diabetic skin conditions.
Source (edited): "http://en.wikipedia.org/wiki/Diabetic_dermopathy"

Diffuse epidermolytic palmoplantar keratoderma

Diffuse epidermolytic palmoplantar keratoderma (also known as "Palmoplantar keratoderma cum degeneratione granulosa Vörner," "Vörner's epidermolytic palmoplantar keratoderma", and "Vörner keratoderma") is one of the most common patterns of palmoplantar keratoderma, an autosomal dominant condition that presents within the first few months of life, characterized by a well-demarcated, symmetric thickening of palms and soles, often with a "dirty" snakeskin appearance sue to underlying epidermolysis.
Source (edited): "http://en.wikipedia.org/wiki/Diffuse_epidermolytic_palmoplantar_keratoderma"

Diffuse nonepidermolytic palmoplantar keratoderma

Diffuse nonepidermolytic palmoplantar keratoderma (also known as "Diffuse orthohyperkeratotic keratoderma," "Hereditary palmoplantar keratoderma," "Keratosis extremitatum progrediens," "Keratosis palmoplantaris diffusa circumscripta," "Tylosis," "Unna–Thost disease", and "Unna–Thost keratoderma") is inherited as an autosomal dominant condition and is present from infancy, characterized by a well-demarcated, symmetric, often "waxy" keratoderma involving the whole of the palms and soles.
Source (edited): "http://en.wikipedia.org/wiki/Diffuse_nonepidermolytic_palmoplantar_keratoderma"

Digitate dermatosis

Digitate dermatosis is a distinct variant of small-plaque parapsoriasis with lesions in the shape of a finger and distributed symmetrically on the flanks.
Source (edited): "http://en.wikipedia.org/wiki/Digitate_dermatosis"

Discoid lupus erythematosus

Discoid lupus erythematosus (DLE) is a chronic skin condition of sores with inflammation and scarring favoring the face, ears, and scalp and at times on other body areas. These lesions develop as a red, inflamed patch with a scaling and crusty appearance. The center areas may appear lighter in color with a rim darker than the normal skin.

Discoid lupus erythematosus can be divided into localized, generalized and childhood discoid lupus erythematosus.

Localized

Localized discoid lupus erythematosus typically presents with skin lesions localized above the neck, with favored sites being the scalp, bridge of nose, cheeks, lower lip, and ears.

Generalized discoid lupus erythematosus

Generalized discoid lupus erythematosus is less common than localized discoid lupus erythematosus, with all degrees of severity being encountered, most often affecting the thorax and upper extremities in addition to the head and neck.

Childhood discoid lupus erythematosus

Childhood discoid lupus erythematosus lacks a female predominance, has a low frequency of photosensitivity, and a higher progression to systemic lupus erythematosus, but in most other respects, the clinical presentation and course is similar to those in adults.

Society and culture

Musician Seal has this skin condition.
Source (edited): "http://en.wikipedia.org/wiki/Discoid_lupus_erythematosus"

Discrete papular lichen myxedematosus

Discrete papular lichen myxedematosus is a skin condition caused by fibroblasts producing abnormally large amounts of mucopolysaccharides characterized by the occurrence of waxy, flesh-colored papules.
Source (edited): "http://en.wikipedia.org/wiki/Discrete_papular_lichen_myxedematosus"

Doucas and Kapetanakis pigmented purpura

Doucas and Kapetanakis pigmented purpura is a skin condition characterized by scaly and eczematous patches, which also have petechiae and hemosiderin staining.

It is also known as "eczematoid purpura" or "eczematoid-like purpura".

It was characterized in 1953.

Source (edited): "http://en.wikipedia.org/wiki/Doucas_and_Kapetanakis_pigmented_purpura"

Drug-induced angioedema

Drug-induced angioedema is a known complication of the use of angiotensin-converting enzyme (ACE) inhibitors and angiotensin II antagonists. The angioedema appears to be dose dependent as it may resolve with decreased dose.

Source (edited): "http://en.wikipedia.org/wiki/Drug-induced_angioedema"

Drug-induced lichenoid reaction

Drug-induced lichenoid reactions (also known as "Lichenoid drug eruption" and "Drug-induced lichen planus") are skin eruptions that occur after ingestion, contact, or inhalation of certain chemicals, with the most common inducers being gold salts, beta blockers, antimalarials, thiazide diuretics, furosemide, spironolactone, and penicillamine. As well as systemic side effects of hypoglycaemic drugs such as Metformin.

Restated, lichenoid drug reactions occur as type IV (delayed) allergic reactions to medications for high blood pressure, heart disease and arthritis. These lichenoid reactions are referred to as lichenoid mucositis (of the mucosa) or dermatitis (of the skin). Allergic reactions to amalgam (metal alloys) dental restorations (fillings) may contribute to the oral lesions identical, both clinically and histologically, to oral lichen planus lesions, and a systematic review found that many of the lesions resolved after the restorations were replaced.

Source (edited): "http://en.wikipedia.org/wiki/Drug-induced_lichenoid_reaction"

Drug-induced pigmentation

Drug-induced pigmentation of the skin may occur as a consequence of drug administration, and the mechanism may be postinflammatory hyperpigmentation in some cases, but frequently is related to actual deposition of the offending drug in the skin.

Source (edited): "http://en.wikipedia.org/wiki/Drug-induced_pigmentation"

Drug-induced pruritus

Drug-induced pruritus is itchiness of the skin caused by medication, a pruritic reaction that is generalized.

Source (edited): "http://en.wikipedia.org/wiki/Drug-induced_pruritus"

Drug-induced pseudolymphoma

Drug-induced pseudolymphoma results from exposure to medications, which results in cutaneous inflammatory patterns that resemble lymphoma, most frequently mycosis fungoides.

Source (edited): "http://en.wikipedia.org/wiki/Drug-induced_pseudolymphoma"

Drug-induced psoriasis

Drug-induced psoriasis may be induced by beta-blockers, lithium, antimalarials, terbinafine, calcium channel blockers, captopril, glyburide, granulocyte colony-stimulating factor, interlukens, interferons, and lipid-lowering drugs.

Source (edited): "http://en.wikipedia.org/wiki/Drug-induced_psoriasis"

Drug-induced purpura

Drug-induced purpura is a skin condition that may be related to platelet destruction, vessel fragility, interference with platelet function, or vasculitis.

Source (edited): "http://en.wikipedia.org/wiki/Drug-induced_purpura"

Drug-induced thrombocytopenic purpura

Drug-induced thrombocytopenic purpura is a skin condition result from a low platelet count due to drug-induced anti-platelet antibodies caused by drugs such as heparin, sulfonamines, digoxin, quinine, and quinidine.

Source (edited): "http://en.wikipedia.org/wiki/Drug-induced_thrombocytopenic_purpura"

Drug-induced ulcer of the lip

A **drug-induced ulcer of the lip** is a condition characterized by painful or tender, well-defined ulcerations of the lip without induration.

Source (edited): "http://en.wikipedia.org/wiki/Drug-induced_ulcer_of_the_lip"

Drug-induced urticaria

Drug-induced urticaria occurs by immunologic and nonimmunologic mechanisms, urticaria most commonly caused by aspirin and NSAIDs.

Source (edited): "http://en.wikipedia.org/wiki/Drug-induced_urticaria"

Dyschromatosis symmetrica hereditaria

Dyschromatosis symmetrica hereditaria (also known as "Reticulate acropigmentation of Dohi," and "Symmetrical dyschromatosis of the extremities") presents primarily in the Japanese, but has also been found to affect individuals from Europe, India, and the Caribbean, characterized by progressively pigmented and depigmented macules, often mixed in a reticulate pattern, concentrated on the dorsal extremities.

Source (edited): "http://en.wikipedia.org/wiki/Dyschromatosis_symmetrica_hereditaria"

Dysplastic nevus syndrome

Dysplastic nevus syndrome (also known as "Familial atypical multiple mole–melanoma (FAMMM) syndrome", "familial melanoma syndrome," and "B-K mole syndrome") is a cutaneous condition described in certain families, and characterized by unusual nevi and multiple inherited melanomas.

Historical background

In 1820 Norris reported the first case of what is now recognized as FAMMM (12). He described a 59-year-old man with melanoma, a high total body mole count, and family history of the same.

Pathology

The histopathologic characteristics of melanoma in FAMMM kindreds are not different from those seen in sporadic cases of melanoma and, thus, are not useful in diagnosing the syndrome. Superficial spreading melanoma (SSM) and nodular melanoma are the most frequently encountered histological melanoma subtypes in patients with CDKN2A mutations, which is consistent with the relative early age of onset.

CDKN2A

The CDKN2A gene is located on chromosome 9p21.3. Two main transcripts, isoforms '1' and '4', each contain three exons and span 7288 and 26740 bp, respectively. They encode proteins of 156 and 173 amino acids; isoform '1' encodes p16(INK4a), while isoform '4' encodes p14(ARF), a protein that is structurally unrelated to p16(INK4) but acts in cell cycle G1 control by stabilizing the tumor suppressor protein p53.

The penetrance for melanoma in kindreds with CDKN2A mutations is estimated at 58% to 92% by 80 years of age and varies with geography. The penetrance in CDKN2A mutation carriers for pancreatic cancer has been estimated to be 17% by 75 years of age. As noted above, there is wide variation in published estimates of the penetrance of CDKN2A mutations.

Management

Screening for melanoma in FAMMM kindreds should begin at age 10 with a baseline total body skin examination including scalp, oral mucosa, genital area, and nail, as family members may develop melanoma in their early teens.

At Mayo Clinic, FAMMM patients with a confirmed mutation and family history of pancreatic cancer are offered screening with either high-resolution pancreatic protocol CT, MRI, or endoscopic ultrasound starting at age 50 or 10 years younger than the earliest family member with pancreas cancer. They are counseled on the lack of evidence-based data to support screening, and on the limitations of our current technology to detect a lesion at a stage amenable to therapy.

Source (edited): "http://en.wikipedia.org/wiki/Dysplastic_nevus_syndrome"

Dystrophic calcinosis cutis

Dystrophic calcinosis cutis is a cutaneous condition characterized by calcification of the skin resulting from the deposition of calcium and phosphorus, and occurs in a preexisting skin lesion of inflammatory process.

Source (edited): "http://en.wikipedia.org/wiki/Dystrophic_calcinosis_cutis"

Ear eczema

Ear eczema may involve the helix, postauricular fold, and external auditory canal, with the most frequently affected site being the external canal, where it is often a manifestation of seborrheic dermatitis or allergic contact dermatitis.

Source (edited): "http://en.wikipedia.org/wiki/Ear_eczema"

Elastosis perforans serpiginosa

Elastosis perforans serpiginosa is a unique perforating disorder characterized by transepidermal elimination of elastic fibers and distinctive clinical lesions, which are serpiginous in distribution and can be associated with specific diseases.

Source (edited): "http://en.wikipedia.org/wiki/Elastosis_perforans_serpiginosa"

Elejalde syndrome

Elejalde syndrome (also known as "Griscelli syndrome type 1") is a rare autosomal recessive syndrome consisting of moderate pigment dilution, profound primary neurologic defects, no immune defects, and hair with metallic silvery sheen.

It is associated with MYO5A.

Source (edited): "http://en.wikipedia.org/wiki/Elejalde_syndrome"

Endemic pemphigus

Endemic pemphigus, also known as **endemic pemphigus foliaceus** and ***fogo selvagem*** (Portuguese for "wildfire"), is a disease that is clinically, histologically, and immunopathologically the same as sporadic pemphigus foliaceus in any individual patient, but that is endemic in the rural areas of Brazil, especially along inland riverbeds.

Source (edited): "http://en.wikipedia.org/wiki/Endemic_pemphigus"

Eosinophilic, polymorphic, and pruritic eruption associated with radiotherapy

Eosinophilic, polymorphic, and pruritic eruption associated with radiotherapy is a skin condition that occurs most often in women receiving cobalt radiotherapy for internal cancer.

Source (edited): "http://en.wikipedia.org/wiki/Eosinophilic,_polymorphic,_and_pruritic_eruption_associated_with_radiotherapy"

Epidermization of the lip

Epidermization of the lip is a condition characterized by relatively smooth leukokeratosis of the lower lip.

Source (edited): "http://en.wikipedia.org/wiki/Epidermization_of_the_lip"

Epidermolysis bullosa acquisita

Epidermolysis bullosa acquisita is a chronic subepidermal blistering disease associated with autoimmunity to type VII collagen within anchoring fibril structures that are located at the dermal-epidermal junction.

Source (edited): "http://en.wikipedia.org/wiki/Epidermolysis_bullosa_acquisita"

Epithelioid blue nevus

Epithelioid blue nevi are a cutaneous condition most commonly seen in patients with the Carney complex.
Source (edited): "http://en.wikipedia.org/wiki/Epithelioid_blue_nevus"

Epulis

Epulis is a term that means any benign lesion situated on the gingiva.
Source (edited): "http://en.wikipedia.org/wiki/Epulis"

Equestrian perniosis

Equestrian perniosis is a skin condition that presents on the lateral thighs of women equestrians who ride on cold damp days.
Source (edited): "http://en.wikipedia.org/wiki/Equestrian_perniosis"

Eruptive lingual papillitis

Eruptive lingual papillitis is a condition characterized by an acute, self-limiting inflammatory stomatitis.
Source (edited): "http://en.wikipedia.org/wiki/Eruptive_lingual_papillitis"

Erythema ab igne

Erythema ab igne (also known as **hot water bottle rash**, **fire stains**, and **toasted skin syndrome**) refers to skin that is reddened due to long-term exposure to infrared radiation.

Erythema ab igne (EAI) is a skin reaction caused by exposure to heat. It was once commonly seen in the elderly who stood or sat closely to open fires or electric heaters. But since Central Heating became widely used it is still sometimes found in people exposed to heat from other sources like heat packs, laptops, and hot water bottles. Overexposure to heat causes a mild red rash that might be described as 'blotchy'. Prolonged and repeated exposure causes a marked redness and colouring of the skin. The skin and underlying tissue may start to thin, and sometimes sores or lesions can develop. Some people may complain of mild itchiness and a burning sensation but often unless a change in pigmentation is seen, it can go unnoticed.

Different types of heat sources can cause this condition such as:

- Repeated application of hot water bottles or heat pads to treat chronic pain, e.g. chronic backache
- Repeated exposure to car heaters or furniture with built-in heaters
- Occupational hazard for silversmiths and jewellers (face exposed to heat), bakers and chefs (arms)

Treatment

The source of heat must be removed. If the area is only mildly affected with slight redness, the condition may resolve by itself in a few months. If the condition is severe and the skin pigmented and atrophic, resolution is unlikely. In this case, there is a possibility that squamous cell carcinomas may form. If there is a persistent sore that doesn't heal or a growing lump within the rash, a skin biopsy should be performed to rule out the possibility of skin cancer. Abnormally pigmented skin may persist for years. Treatment with topical tretinoin or laser may improve the appearance.

It may also be seen in people with hypothyroidism, lymphoedema.
Source (edited): "http://en.wikipedia.org/wiki/Erythema_ab_igne"

Erythema dyschromicum perstans

Erythema dyschromicum perstans (also known as "Ashy dermatosis," and "Dermatosis cinecienta") is a skin condition with age of onset almost always before 40 years old, characterized by skin lesions that are usually symmetrical and generalized.
Source (edited): "http://en.wikipedia.org/wiki/Erythema_dyschromicum_perstans"

Erythema elevatum diutinum

Erythema elevatum diutinum is a form of vasculitis.

It has been described as a paraneoplastic syndrome.

Source (edited): "http://en.wikipedia.org/wiki/Erythema_elevatum_diutinum"

Erythema gyratum repens

Erythema gyratum repens (also known as "Gammel's disease") is a figurate erythema that is rapidly moving and usually a cancer marker.

Source (edited): "http://en.wikipedia.org/wiki/Erythema_gyratum_repens"

Erythema multiforme

Erythema multiforme is a skin condition of unknown cause, possibly mediated by deposition of immune complex (mostly IgM) in the superficial microvasculature of the skin and oral mucous membrane that usually follows an infection or drug exposure. It is a common disorder, with peak incidence in the second and third decades of life.

Presentation

The condition varies from a mild, self-limited rash (E. multiforme minor) to a severe, life-threatening form known as **erythema multiforme major** (or **erythema multiforme majus**) that also involves mucous membranes. This severe form may be related to Stevens-Johnson syndrome. The mild form is far more common than the severe form. Diagnosis is confirmed by biopsy.

The mild form usually presents with mildly itchy, pink-red blotches, symmetrically arranged and starting on the extremities. It often takes on the classical "target lesion" appearance, with a pink-red ring around a pale center. Resolution within 7–10 days is the norm.

Individuals with persistent (chronic) erythema multiforme will often have a sore form at an injury site, eg. a minor scratch or abrasion, within a week. Irritation or even pressure from clothing will cause the erythema sore to continue to expand along its margins for weeks or months, long after the original sore at the center heals. ,,,,

Causes

The most common predisposing infection is Herpes simplex, but bacterial infections (commonly *Mycoplasma*) and fungal diseases are also implicated. Herpes simplex virus suppression and even prophylaxis (with acyclovir) has been shown to prevent recurrent erythema multiforme eruption.

Other causes include drug reactions, most commonly to sulfa drugs, phenytoin, barbiturates, penicillin, and allopurinol, or a host of internal ailments.

The human form of orf can also cause erythema multiforme.

Persistent (chronic) erythema multiforme has been linked to ingestion of benzoates in both natural and artificial forms, including benzoic acid, which occurs naturally in some fruit, and sodium benzoate, a common food preservative.

Treatment

Erythema multiforme is frequently self-limiting and requires no treatment. The appropriateness of glucocorticoid therapy can be uncertain, because it is difficult to determine if the course will be self-limiting.

Source (edited): "http://en.wikipedia.org/wiki/Erythema_multiforme"

Erythema multiforme minor

Erythema multiforme minor (also known as "Herpes simplex-associated erythema multiforme") is a skin condition associated with a preceding herpetic infection, characterized by skin lesions that begin as sharply marginated, erythematous macules, which then become raised and develop a target-like appearance.

Erythema multiforme minor is sometimes divided into papular and vesiulobullous forms.

Source (edited): "http://en.wikipedia.org/wiki/Erythema_multiforme_minor"

Erythema toxicum neonatorum

Erythema toxicum neonatorum (also known as "Erythema toxicum," and "Toxic erythema of the newborn") is a common rash in neonates. It appears in up to half of newborns carried to term, usually between day 2-5 after birth.

Erythema toxicum is characterized by blotchy red spots on the skin with overlying white or yellow papules or pustules. These lesions may be few or numerous. The eruption typically resolves within a few days.

Cause

The cause of erythema toxicum is unknown.

Hypersensitivity to detergents in bedsheets and clothing is sometimes suspected, but the connection remains unproven.

It is thought to be a benign condition that causes no discomfort to the infant. The rash will generally disappear spontaneously in about 2 weeks.

Presentation

The rash is composed of small papular lesions, each on a separate reddened base.

Diagnosis

At times the appearance can raise concern that the rash could be due to herpes simplex; however, the latter generally has a more clustered and vesicular appearance.

In uncertain cases, a scraping of a lesion can be done and the fluid examined under the microscope. Herpes lesions will have a positive direct fluorescent antibody test. The fluid from erythema toxicum lesions will show many eosinophils.

Treatment

Because the eruption is transient and self-limiting, no treatment is indicated
Source (edited): "http://en.wikipedia.org/wiki/Erythema_toxicum_neonatorum"

Erythrocyanosis crurum

Erythrocyanosis crurum is a skin condition, a variant of acrocyanosis caused by chronic exposure to cold.
Source (edited): "http://en.wikipedia.org/wiki/Erythrocyanosis_crurum"

Erythroderma

Erythroderma (also known as "Exfoliative dermatitis," "Dermatitis exfoliativa," and "Red man syndrome") is an inflammatory skin disease with erythema and scaling that affects nearly the entire cutaneous surface.

In ICD-10, a distinction is made between "exfoliative dermatitis" at L26, and "erythroderma" at L53.9.

Historical aspects

The classification of exfoliative dermatitis into Wilson-Brocq (chronic relapsing), Hebra or pityriasis rubra (progressive), and Savill (self-limited) types may have had historical value, but it currently lacks pathophysiologic or clinical utility.

Causes

Erythroderma is generalized exfoliative dermatitis, which involves 90% or more of the patient's skin. The most common cause of erythroderma is exacerbation of an underlying skin disease, such as psoriasis, contact dermatitis, seborrheic dermatitis, lichen planus, pityriasis rubra pilaris or a drug reaction. Primary erythroderma is less frequent and is usually seen in cases of cutaneous T-cell lymphoma, in particular in Sézary's disease.

The most common causes of exfoliative dermatitis are best remembered by the mnemonic device ID-SCALP. . The causes and their frequencies are as follows:

- Idiopathic - 30%
- Drug allergy - 28%
- Seborrheic dermatitis - 2%
- Contact dermatitis - 3%
- Atopic dermatitis - 10%
- Lymphoma and leukemia - 14%
- Psoriasis - 8%

Differential diagnosis in patients with erythroderma may be difficult.

Treatment

The treatment is dependent on the cause.
Source (edited): "http://en.wikipedia.org/wiki/Erythroderma"

Erythrodermic sarcoidosis

Erythrodermic sarcoidosis is a cutaneous condition and very rare form of sarcoidosis.
Source (edited): "http://en.wikipedia.org/wiki/Erythrodermic_sarcoidosis"

Erythrotelangiectatic rosacea

Erythrotelangiectatic rosacea (also known as "Erythematotelangiectatic rosacea" and "Vascular rosacea") is characterized by prominent history of prolonged (over ten minutes) flushing reaction to various stimuli, such as emotional stress, hot drinks, alcohol, spicy foods, exercise, cold or hot weather, or hot baths and showers.
Source (edited): "http://en.wikipedia.org/wiki/Erythrotelangiectatic_rosacea"

Essential dermatitis

Essential dermatitis is an idiopathic inflammation of the skin that does not fit the picture of other well defined conditions (such as atopic or contact dermatitis) and is a diagnosis of exclusion.
Source (edited): "http://en.wikipedia.org/wiki/Essential_dermatitis"

Excoriated acne

Excoriated acne (also known as "Picker's acne" or "Acne excoriée des jeunes filles") is a mild acne accompanied by extensive excoriations.
Source (edited): "http://en.wikipedia.org/wiki/Excoriated_acne"

Exudative hyponychial dermatitis

Exudative hyponychial dermatitis is a nail toxicity common during chemotherapy for breast cancer, especially if docetaxel is the chemotherapeutic regimen.
Source (edited): "http://en.wikipedia.org/wiki/Exudative_hyponychial_dermatitis"

Eyelid dermatitis

Eyelid dermatitis is commonly related to atopic dermatitis or allergic contact dermatitis. Volatile substances, tosylamide, epoxy hardeners, insect sprays, and lemon peel oil may be implicated, with many cases of eyelid contact dermatitis being caused by substances transferred by the hands to the eyelids.
Source (edited): "http://en.wikipedia.org/wiki/Eyelid_dermatitis"

Factitial lymphedema

Factitial lymphedema (also known as "Hysterical edema") is a skin condition produced by wrapping an elastic bandage, cord, or shirt around an extremity, and/or holding the extremity in a dependent and immobile state.
Source (edited): "http://en.wikipedia.org/wiki/Factitial_lymphedema"

Factitial panniculitis

Factitial panniculitis is a skin condition characterized by inflammation of the subcutaneous fat that may be induced by the injection of organic materials, povidone, feces, saliva, vaginal fluid, and oils.
Source (edited): "http://en.wikipedia.org/wiki/Factitial_panniculitis"

Factitious dermatitis

Factitious dermatitis (also known as "Dermatitis artefacta") is a form of factitious disorder in which patients will intentionally feign symptoms and produce signs of disease in an attempt to assume the patient role.
Source (edited): "http://en.wikipedia.org/wiki/Factitious_dermatitis"

Familial acanthosis nigricans

Familial acanthosis nigricans (also known as "Acanthosis nigricans type II") is an exceedingly rare type of acanthosis nigricans that is present at birth or develop during childhood.

Gallery

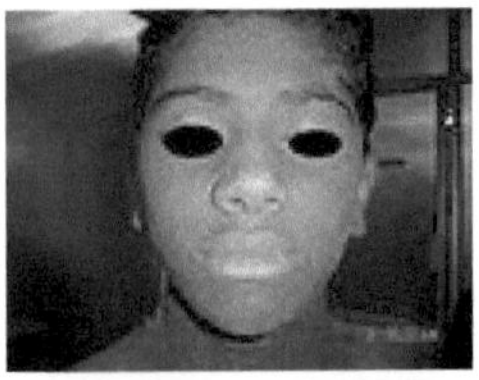

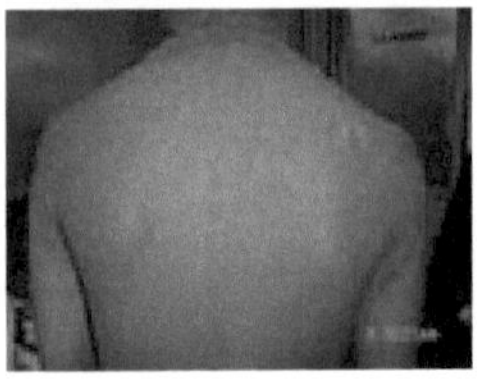

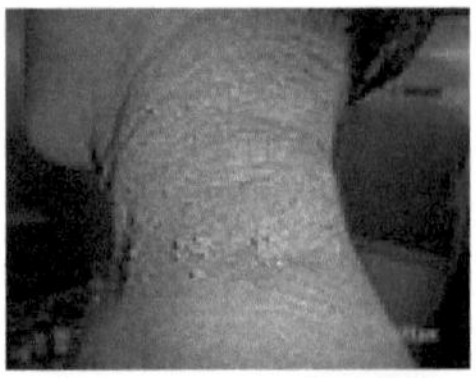

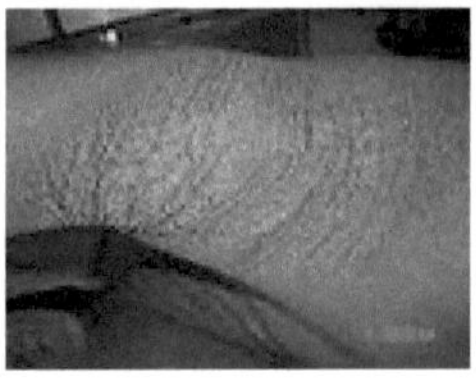

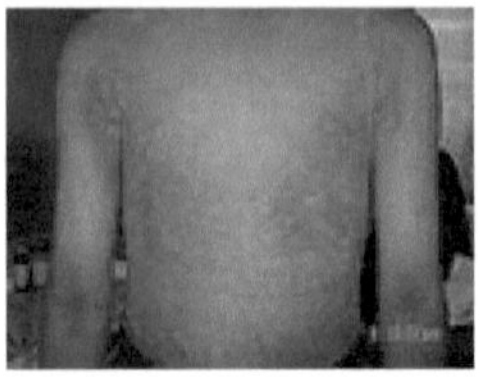

Source (edited): "http://en.wikipedia.org/wiki/Familial_acanthosis_nigricans"

Familial apoprotein CII deficiency

Familial apoprotein CII deficiency is a condition caused by a lack of lipoprotein lipase activator.
Source (edited): "http://en.wikipedia.org/wiki/Familial_apoprotein_CII_deficiency"

Familial cold urticaria

Familial cold urticaria (also properly known as **familial cold autoinflammatory syndrome, FCAS**) is an autosomal dominant condition characterized by rash, conjunctivitis, fever/chills and arthralgias elicited by exposure to cold - sometimes temperatures below 22°C (72°F).

It has been mapped to CIAS1 and is a slightly milder member of the disease family including Muckle–Wells syndrome and NOMID. It is rare and is estimated as having a prevalence of 1 per million people and mainly affects Americans and Europeans.

FCAS is one of the cryopyrin-associated periodic syndromes (CAPS) caused by mutations in the CIAS1/NALP3 (aka NLRP3) gene at location 1q44.

The effect of FCAS on the quality of life of patients is far reaching. A survey of patients in the United States in 2008 found, "To cope with their underlying disease and to try to avoid symptomatic, painful, flares patients reported limiting their work, school, family, and social activities. Seventy-eight percent of survey participants described an impact of the disease on their work, including absenteeism and impaired job advancement; frequently they quit their job as a consequence of their disease".

Treatment using anakinra (Kineret) has been shown effective for FCAS although this does mean daily injections of the immunosuppressant into an area such as the lower abdomen. The monoclonal antibody canakinumab (Ilaris) is also used.
Source (edited): "http://en.wikipedia.org/wiki/Familial_cold_urticaria"

Familial dysbetalipoproteinemia

Familial dysbetalipoproteinemia (also known as "Broad beta disease" and "Remnant removal disease") is a condition characterized by increased LDL, triglyceride, and cholesterol levels, and decreased HDL levels. The condition is caused by a deficiency in apolipoprotein E that serves as a ligand for chylomicron and IDL receptors in the liver: The normal ApoE turns into the defective ApoE2 form.
Source (edited): "http://en.wikipedia.org/wiki/Familial_dysbetalipoproteinemia"

Familial hypertriglyceridemia

Familial hypertriglyceridemia is an autosomal dominant condition occurring in 1-2% of the population. Triglyceride levels, but not cholesterol, are elevated as a result of excess hepatic production of VLDL or heterozygous LPL deficiency. Unlike familial hypercholesterolemia, there is no association with premature coronary disease. However, affected individuals are at risk for chylomicronemia syndrome, characterized by elevated chylomicrons in the blood.
Source (edited): "http://en.wikipedia.org/wiki/Familial_hypertriglyc-

eridemia"

Familial partial lipodystrophy

Familial partial lipodystrophy (also known as "Köbberling–Dunnigan syndrome") is an autosomal dominant skin condition characterized by the loss of subcutaneous fat.

Type 1 is believed to be underdiagnosed.

Source (edited): "http://en.wikipedia.org/wiki/Familial_partial_lipodystrophy"

Familial progressive hyperpigmentation

Familial progressive hyperpigmentation is characterized by patches of hyperpigmentation, present at birth, which increase in size and number with age.

Source (edited): "http://en.wikipedia.org/wiki/Familial_progressive_hyperpigmentation"

Favre–Racouchot syndrome

Favre–Racouchot syndrome (also known as "Favre–Racouchot disease," and "Nodular cutaneous elastosis with cysts and comedones") is a disorder consisting of multiple open comedones that occurs in skin damaged by sunlight, especially under and lateral of the eyes. The comedones are widened openings for hair follicles and sebaceous glands filled with horny material.

Source (edited): "http://en.wikipedia.org/wiki/Favre%E2%80%93Racouchot_syndrome"

Fibrinolysis syndrome

Fibrinolysis syndrome (also known as "Defibrinating syndrome," and "Hypofibrinogenemia") is characterized by an acute hemorrhagic state brought about by inability of the blood to clot, with massive hemorrhages into the skin producing blackish, purplish swellings and sloughing.

Source (edited): "http://en.wikipedia.org/wiki/Fibrinolysis_syndrome"

Fixed drug reaction

Fixed drug reactions are common and so named because they recur at the same site with each exposure to a particular medication. Medications inducing fixed drug eruptions are usually those taken intermittently.

Source (edited): "http://en.wikipedia.org/wiki/Fixed_drug_reaction"

Focal acral hyperkeratosis

Focal acral hyperkeratosis (also known as "Acrokeratoelastoidosis lichenoides," and "Degenerative collagenous plaques of the hand") is a late-onset keratoderma, inherited as an autosomal dominant condition, characterized by oval or polygonal crateriform papules developing along the border of the hands, feet, and wrists.

It is considered similar to Costa acrokeratoelastoidosis.

Source (edited): "http://en.wikipedia.org/wiki/Focal_acral_hyperkeratosis"

Food-induced purpura

Food-induced purpura is a skin condition that may result from ingestion of tartrazine dye, benzoates, and food containing Escherichia coli O157:H7.

Source (edited): "http://en.wikipedia.org/wiki/Food-induced_purpura"

Fracture blister

Fracture blisters occur on skin overlying a fractured bone, and fractures complicated by the development of overlying blisters remain a clinical dilemma in orthopedics.
Source (edited): "http://en.wikipedia.org/wiki/Fracture_blister"

Friction blister

Friction blisters are a skin condition that may occur at sites of combined pressure and friction, and may be enhanced by heat and moisture, characterized by vesicles or bullae.
Source (edited): "http://en.wikipedia.org/wiki/Friction_blister"

Galli–Galli disease

Galli–Galli disease is a rare inherited condition that has close resemblance clinically to Dowling-Degos' disease, but is histologically distinct, characterized by skin lesions that are 1- to 2-mm slightly keratotic red to dark brown papules which are focally confluent in a reticulate pattern. The disease is also characterized by slowly progressive and disfiguring reticulate hyperpigmentation of the flexures, clinically and histopathologically diagnostic for Dowling-Degos disease but also associated with suprabasal, nondyskeratotic acantholysis.
Source (edited): "http://en.wikipedia.org/wiki/Galli%E2%80%93Galli_disease"

Galvanic urticaria

Galvanic urticaria has been described after exposure to a galvanic device used to treat hyperhidrosis.
Source (edited): "http://en.wikipedia.org/wiki/Galvanic_urticaria"

Generalized eruptive histiocytoma

Generalized eruptive histiocytoma (also known as "Eruptive histiocytoma," and "Generalized eruptive histiocytosis") is a rare cutaneous condition characterized by widespread, erythematous, essentially symmetrical papules, particularly involving the trunk and proximal extremities.
Source (edited): "http://en.wikipedia.org/wiki/Generalized_eruptive_histiocytoma"

Generalized erythema

Generalized erythema is a skin condition that may be caused by medications, bacterial toxins, or viral infections.
Source (edited): "http://en.wikipedia.org/wiki/Generalized_erythema"

Generalized granuloma annulare

Generalized granuloma annulare is a skin condition of unknown cause, tending to affect women in the fifth and sixth decades, presenting as a diffuse but symmetrical, papular or annular eruption of more than ten skin lesions, and often hundreds.

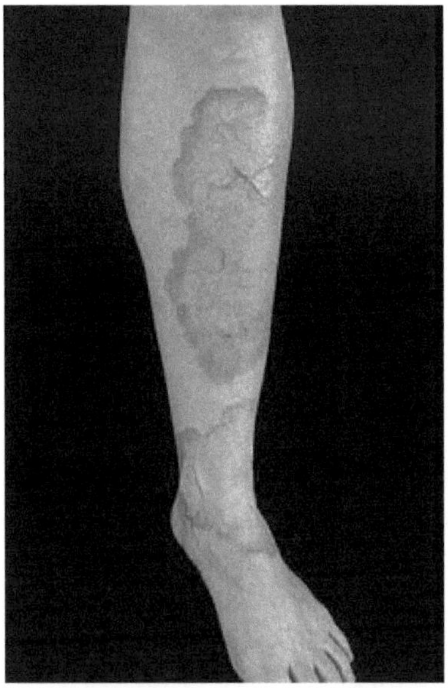

Generalized granuloma annulare

Source (edited): "http://en.wikipedia.org/wiki/Generalized_granuloma_annulare"

Generalized lentiginosis

Generalized lentiginosis is a cutaneous condition that will occasionally present without other associated abnormalities. It may be caused by carney complex, LEOPARD syndrome or Peutz–Jeghers syndrome.

Source (edited): "http://en.wikipedia.org/wiki/Generalized_lentiginosis"

Generalized morphea

Generalized morphea is characterized by widespread indurated plaques and pigmentary changes, sometimes associated with muscle atrophy, but without visceral involvement.

Source (edited): "http://en.wikipedia.org/wiki/Generalized_morphea"

Giant pigmented nevus

Giant pigmented nevus (also known as "Bathing trunk nevus," "Congenital nevomelanocytic nevus," "Garment nevus," "Giant hairy nevus", and "Nevus pigmentosus et pilosus") is a cutaneous condition characterized by a large, darkly pigmented hairy patches.

Source (edited): "http://en.wikipedia.org/wiki/Giant_pigmented_nevus"

Glandular rosacea

In **Glandular rosacea**, men with thick sebaceous skin predominate, a disease in which the papules are edematous, the pustules often 0.5 to 1.0cm in size, with nodulocystic lesions often present.

Source (edited): "http://en.wikipedia.org/wiki/Glandular_rosacea"

Gnathophyma

Gnathophyma involves swelling of the chin.

Source (edited): "http://en.wikipedia.org/wiki/Gnathophyma"

Gougerot–Blum syndrome

Gougerot–Blum syndrome (also known as "Pigmented purpuric lichenoid dermatitis," and "Pigmented purpuric lichenoid dermatitis of Gougerot and Blum") is a variant of Pigmented purpuric dermatitis, a skin condition characterized by minute, rust-colored to violaceous, lichenoid papules that tend to fuse into plaques of various hues. Relative to other variants, it is characterized clinically by a male predominance, puritis, with a predilication for the legs, and histologically, it features a densely cellular lichenoid infiltrate.

It was characterized in 1925.

Source (edited): "http://en.wikipedia.org/wiki/Gougerot%E2%80%93Blum_syndrome"

Gouty panniculitis

Gouty panniculitis is a skin condition characterized by inflammation of the subcutaneous fat caused by deposition of uric acid crystals.

Source (edited): "http://en.wikipedia.org/wiki/Gouty_panniculitis"

Gram-negative rosacea

Gram-negative rosacea is a cutaneous condition that clinically looks like stage II or III rosacea.

Source (edited): "http://en.wikipedia.org/wiki/Gram-negative_rosacea"

Granuloma annulare in HIV disease

Granuloma annulare in HIV disease is a skin condition characterized typically by papular and generalized skin lesions.

Source (edited): "http://en.wikipedia.org/wiki/Granuloma_annulare_in_HIV_disease"

Granuloma faciale

Granuloma faciale (GF) is an uncommon benign chronic skin disease of unknown origin characterized by single or multiple cutaneous nodules, usually occurring over the face. Occasionally, extrafacial involvement is noted, most often on sun-exposed areas.

History

Lever and Leeper first recognized GF as a distinct entity in 1950. Pinkus' group suggested the name granuloma faciale that same year.

Differential diagnosis

The disease mimics many other dermatoses and can be confused with conditions, such as sarcoidosis, discoid lupus erythematosus, mycosis fungoides, and fixed drug eruption.

Source (edited): "http://en.wikipedia.org/wiki/Granuloma_faciale"

Granuloma multiforme

Granuloma multiforme is a cutaneous condition most commonly seen in central Africa, and rarely elsewhere, characterized by skin lesions that are on the upper trunk and arms in sun-exposed areas.

Source (edited): "http://en.wikipedia.org/wiki/Granuloma_multiforme"

Granulomatous facial dermatitis

Granulomatous facial dermatitis is found in patients with persistent facial erythema involving one or more convex surfaces of the face, with lesions that show granulomatous reaction histologically.

Source (edited): "http://en.wikipedia.org/wiki/Granulomatous_facial_dermatitis"

Granulomatous perioral dermatitis

Granulomatous perioral dermatitis is a cutaneous condition found in otherwise healthy prepubertal children, in which there is a profusion of grouped papules on the perioral, periocular, and perinasal areas.

Source (edited): "http://en.wikipedia.org/wiki/Granulomatous_perioral_dermatitis"

Granulomatous slack skin

Granulomatous slack skin (GSS) is a rare cutaneous condition, a variant of lymphoma that typically presents in middle aged adults.

Source (edited): "http://en.wikipedia.org/wiki/Granulomatous_slack_skin"

Griscelli syndrome type 2

Griscelli syndrome type 2 (also known as "Partial albinism with immunodeficiency") is a rare autosomal recessive syndrome characterized by variable pigmentary dilution, hair with silvery metallic sheen, frequent pyogenic infections, neutropenia, and thrombocytopenia.

Source (edited): "http://en.wikipedia.org/wiki/Griscelli_syndrome_type_2"

Griscelli syndrome type 3

Griscelli syndrome type 3 is a disorder of melanosome transport presenting initially with hypopigmentation.

Source (edited): "http://en.wikipedia.org/wiki/Griscelli_syndrome_type_3"

Guttate psoriasis

Guttate psoriasis (also known as "Eruptive psoriasis") presents as small (0.5-1.5 cm in diameter) lesions over the upper trunk and proximal extremities, a form characterized by early age of onset and as such is found frequently in young adults. Guttate psoriasis is classically triggered by a bacterial infection, usually an upper respiratory tract infection.

Source (edited): "http://en.wikipedia.org/wiki/Guttate_psoriasis"

HAIR-AN syndrome

HAIR-AN syndrome consists of hyperandrogenism, insulin resistance, and acanthosis nigricans.

It is a subset of polycystic ovary syndrome.

Source (edited): "http://en.wikipedia.org/wiki/HAIR-AN_syndrome"

HIV-associated lipodystrophy

HIV-associated lipodystrophy is a condition characterized by loss of subcutaneous fat associated with infection with HIV.

Cause

The exact mechanism of HIV-associated lipodystrophy is not fully elucidated. However, on the one hand, it is believed to be caused by anti-retroviral medications. Lipodystrophy seems to be mainly due to HIV-1 protease inhibitors. Interference with lipid metabolism is postulated as pathophysiology. Also, the development of lipodystrophy is associated with specific nucleoside reverse transcriptase inhibitors (NRTI). Mitochondrial toxicity is postulated to be involved in the pathogenesis associated with NRTI.

On the other hand, there is evidence that HIV-1 infection on its own contributes to the development of the lipodystrophic phenotype by interfering with some key genes of adipocyte differentiation and mitochondrial function on patients which have not received antiretroviral treatment.

Presentations include

HIV-associated lipodystrophy commonly presents with fat loss in face, buttocks, arms and legs.

There is also fat *accumulation* caused by these drugs in various body parts. Patients often present with "buffalo hump" like fat deposits in their upper backs. Breast sizes of patients (both male and female) tends to increase. In addition, patients develop abdominal obesity, commonly described as a "beer gut".

Prognosis

Reversion of lipodystrophy does not occur after withdrawal of protease inhibitors.

Source (edited): "http://en.wikipedia.org/wiki/HIV-associated_lipodystrophy"

HIV disease-related drug reaction

HIV disease-related drug reactions present in HIV-infected patients, especially those with helper T-cell counts between 25 and 200, immunosuppression that increases the risk for the development of adverse reactions to medications.

Source (edited): "http://en.wikipedia.org/wiki/HIV_disease-related_drug_reaction"

Haber syndrome

Haber syndrome is a cutaneous disorder of hyperpigmentation characterized by reticulated pigmentation of the person's skin. A rare genodermatosis, its key features include "rosacea-like facial eruption[,] reticulated hyperpigmentation of major flexures, comedones on the back and neck, and pitted facial scars."

Source (edited): "http://en.wikipedia.org/wiki/Haber_syndrome"

Halogen acne

Halogen acne is caused by iodides and bromides that induce an acneiform eruption similar to that observed with steroids.

Source (edited): "http://en.wikipedia.org/wiki/Halogen_acne"

Hand eczema

Hand eczema presents on the palms and soles, and may sometimes be difficult or impossible to differentiate from atopic dermatitis, allergic contact dermatitis, and psoriasis, which also commonly involve the hands. Even a biopsy of all these conditions may not result in a definitive diagnosis, as all three conditions may demonstrate spongiosis and crusting on the hands.

Source (edited): "http://en.wikipedia.org/wiki/Hand_eczema"

Heat urticaria

Heat urticaria presents within five minutes after the skin has been exposed to heat above 43 degrees Celsius (109.4 degrees Fahrenheit), with the exposed area becoming burned, stinging, and turning red, swollen, and indurated.

Source (edited): "http://en.wikipedia.org/wiki/Heat_urticaria"

Hematopoietic ulcer

Hematopoietic ulcers are those occurring with sickle cell anemia, Cooley anemia, congenital hemolytic anemia, polycythemia vera, thrombocytopenic purpura, macroglobulinemia, and cryoglobulinemia.

Source (edited): "http://en.wikipedia.org/wiki/Hematopoietic_ulcer"

Hemosiderin hyperpigmentation

Hemosiderin hyperpigmentation is pigmentation due to deposits of hemosiderin, and occurs in purpura, hemochromotosis, hemorrhagic diseases, and stasis dermatitis.

Source (edited): "http://en.wikipedia.org/wiki/Hemosiderin_hyperpigmentation"

Hennekam syndrome

Hennekam syndrome also known as **Hennekam lymphangiectasia–lymphedema syndrome** and **intestinal lymphagiectasia–lymphedema–mental retardation syndrome** is an autosomal recessive disorder consisting of intestinal lymphangiectasia, facial anomalies, peripheral lymphedema, and mild to moderate levels of growth and mental retardation.

It is also known as "lymphedema-lymphangiectasia-mental retardation syndrome".

It may be associated with CCBE1.

Source (edited): "http://en.wikipedia.org/wiki/Hennekam_syndrome"

Hepatitis-associated lichen planus

Hepatitis-associated lichen planus is a skin condition that has been associated with three liver conditions: hepatitis C viral infection, hepatitis B immunization, and primary biliary cirrhosis.

Source (edited): "http://en.wikipedia.org/wiki/Hepatitis-associated_lichen_planus"

Hereditary progressive mucinous histiocytosis

Hereditary progressive mucinous histiocytosis is an autosomal dominant or X-linked hereditary described on in women.

Source (edited): "http://en.wikipedia.org/wiki/Hereditary_progressive_mucinous_histiocytosis"

Heredofamilial amyloidosis

Heredofamilial amyloidosis is an inherited condition that may be characterized by systemic or localized deposition of amyloid in body tissues.

Source (edited): "http://en.wikipedia.org/wiki/Heredofamilial_amyloidosis"

Hyaluronidase deficiency

Hyaluronidase deficiency (also known as "Mucopolysaccharidosis type IX") is a condition caused by mutations in HYAL1, and characterized by multiple soft-tissue masses.

Source (edited): "http://en.wikipedia.org/wiki/Hyaluronidase_deficiency"

Hydroa vacciniforme

Hydroa vacciniforme (also known as "Bazin's hydroa vacciniforme") is a skin condition, a very rare, chronic photodermatitis with onset in childhood. It is seen in children under 10 years of age,and it disappears at puberty. It starts after being exposed to the summer sun , it starts as an vesicular eruption then becomes umbilicated and in the end there is a chickenpox-like scar. it is seen on the nose,cheeks,ears,dorsum of the hand,and arms (places that are most exposed to light).

Source (edited): "http://en.wikipedia.org/wiki/Hydroa_vacciniforme"

Hydroxyethyl starch-induced pruritus

Hydroxyethyl starch-induced pruritus is an intense itching, lasting for as long as one year, occurring following hydroxyethyl starch intravenous infusion for vascular insufficiency.

Source (edited): "http://en.wikipedia.org/wiki/Hydroxyethyl_starch-induced_pruritus"

Hydroxyurea dermopathy

Hydroxyurea dermopathy is caused by chronic use of hydroxyurea for chronic myelogenous leukemia, thrombocytopenia, or psoriasis, and presents with skin lesions characteristic of dermatomyositis.

Source (edited): "http://en.wikipedia.org/wiki/Hydroxyurea_dermopathy"

Hyperkeratotic hand dermatitis

Hyperkeratotic hand dermatitis presents with hyperkeratotic, fissure-prone, erythematous areas of the middle or proximal palm, and the volar surfaces of the fingers may also be involved.

Source (edited): "http://en.wikipedia.org/wiki/Hyperkeratotic_hand_dermatitis"

Hypertrophic lichen planus

Hypertrophic lichen planus (also known as "Lichen planus verrucosus") usually occurs on the extremities, especially the shin and interphalangeal joints, and tends to be the most pruritic variant of lichen planus.

Source (edited): "http://en.wikipedia.org/wiki/Hypertrophic_lichen_planus"

Hypopigmented sarcoidosis

Hypopigmented sarcoidosis is a cutaneous condition characterized by areas of hypopigmented skin. It is usually diagnosed in darkly pigmented races and may be the earliest sign of sarcoidosis.

Source (edited): "http://en.wikipedia.org/wiki/Hypopigmented_sarcoidosis"

Iatrogenic calcinosis cutis

Iatrogenic calcinosis cutis is a cutaneous condition characterized by calcification of the skin resulting from the deposition of calcium and phosphorus inadvertently introduced by a medical procedure.

Source (edited): "http://en.wikipedia.org/wiki/Iatrogenic_calcinosis_cutis"

Ichthyosiform sarcoidosis

Ichthyosiform sarcoidosis is a cutaneous condition resembling ichthyosis vulgaris or acquired ichthyosis, with fine scaling usually on the distal extremities, by caused by sarcoidosis.

Source (edited): "http://en.wikipedia.org/wiki/Ichthyosiform_sarcoidosis"

Ichthyosis acquisita

Ichthyosis acquisita (or "acquired ichthyosis") is a disorder clinically and histologically similar to ichthyosis vulgaris.

Associated conditions

The development of ichthyosis in adulthood can be a manifestation of systemic disease, and it has been described in association with malignancies, drugs, endocrine and metabolic disease, HIV, infection, and autoimmune conditions.

It usually is associated with people who have Hodgkin's disease but it is also occurs in people with mycosis fungoides, other malignant sarcomas, Kaposi's sarcoma and visceral carcinomas. It can occur in people suffering from leprosy, AIDS, tuberculosis, and typhoid fever.

Source (edited): "http://en.wikipedia.org/wiki/Ichthyosis_acquisita"

Ichthyosis en confetti

Ichthyosis en confetti, also known as **ichthyosis with confetti**. **congenital reticular ichthyosiform erythroderma (CRIE)** and **ichthyosis variegata**, is a very rare form of congenital ichthyosis in which healthy patches of normal skin co-exist within the abnormal skin areas. It has been hypothesized that this is the result of a combination of mitotic recombination and natural selection within the skin. Choate et. al. have shown that mutations in a gene called *keratin-10* cause this disorder. They show that mutant keratin 10 accumulates in the nucleolus, a sub-nuclear structure, rather than within cellular intermedite filaments like the wild-type protein. It has been speculated that the presence of mutantkeratin 10 results in increased rates of mitotic recombination, thus in effect leading the disease to effect its own partial "cure".

Source (edited): "http://en.wikipedia.org/wiki/Ichthyosis_en_confetti"

Id reaction

Id reactions (also known as "Disseminated eczema," and "Generalized eczema") present with a variety of infectious disorders, often occurring in response to an inflammatory tinea of the feet, resulting in an eczematous dermatitis. Id reactions are frequently unresponsive to corticosteroid therapy, but clear when the focus of infection or infestation is treated.

Source (edited): "http://en.wikipedia.org/wiki/Id_reaction"

Idiopathic eruptive macular pigmentation

Idiopathic eruptive macular pigmentation is a skin condition developing in young persons, with an average age of 11, characterized by asymptomatic widespread brown to gray macules of up to several centimeters in diameter on the neck, trunk, and proximal extremities.

Source (edited): "http://en.wikipedia.org/wiki/Idiopathic_eruptive_macular_pigmentation"

Idiopathic facial aseptic granuloma

Idiopathic facial aseptic granuloma is a cutaneous condition characterized by a chronic, painless, solitary nodule, reminiscent of an acne nodule, appearing on the cheeks of young children.

Source (edited): "http://en.wikipedia.org/wiki/Idiopathic_facial_aseptic_granuloma"

Idiopathic guttate hypomelanosis

Idiopathic guttate hypomelanosis (also known as "Leukopathia symmetrica progressiva") is a very common acquired disorder that affects women more frequently than men, presenting with skin lesions that occur chiefly on the skins and forearms, suggesting sun exposure may play a role.

Source (edited): "http://en.wikipedia.org/wiki/Idiopathic_guttate_hypomelanosis"

Idiopathic scrotal calcinosis

Idiopathic scrotal calcinosis (also known as "Idiopathic calcified nodules of the scrotum") is a cutaneous condition characterized by calcification of the skin resulting from the deposition of calcium and phosphorus occurring on the scrotum.

Treatment may involve surgery.

The cause is not well defined.

Source (edited): "http://en.wikipedia.org/wiki/Idiopathic_scrotal_calcinosis"

Immunodeficiency with hyperimmunoglobulin M

Immunodeficiency with hyperimmunoglobulin M is a rare disorder characterized by recurrent infections, low or absent IgG, IgE, and IgA levels, and normal or elevated levels of IgM and IgD.

Source (edited): "http://en.wikipedia.org/wiki/Immunodeficiency_with_hyperimmunoglobulin_M"

Indeterminate cell histiocytosis

Indeterminate cell histiocytosis is a cutaneous condition felt to be caused by dermal precursors of Langerhans cells.

Source (edited): "http://en.wikipedia.org/wiki/Indeterminate_cell_histiocytosis"

Infantile acne

Infantile acne is a cutaneous condition that presents at 3 to 6 months of age.

Source (edited): "http://en.wikipedia.org/wiki/Infantile_acne"

Infantile acropustulosis

Infantile acropustulosis (also known as "Acropustulosis of infancy") is an intensely itchy vesicopustular eruption of the hands and feet.

Involvement of scabies has been suggested.

Source (edited): "http://en.wikipedia.org/wiki/Infantile_acropustulosis"

Inherited patterned lentiginosis in black persons

Inherited patterned lentiginosis in black persons is a cutaneous condition inherited in an autosomal dominant fashion, presenting in infancy or early childhood.

Source (edited): "http://en.wikipedia.org/wiki/Inherited_patterned_lentiginosis_in_black_persons"

Injection site reaction

Injection site reactions are allergic reactions that result in cutaneous necrosis that may occur at sites of medication injection, typically presenting in one of two forms, (1) those associated with intravenous infusion or (2) those related to intramuscular injection. Intra muscular injections may produce a syndrome called livedo dermatitis.

Source (edited): "http://en.wikipedia.org/wiki/Injection_site_reaction"

Ink spot lentigo

Ink spot lentigo (also known as "Sunburn lentigo") is a cutaneous condition characterized by skin lesions commonly occurring on the shoulders.

Source (edited): "http://en.wikipedia.org/wiki/Ink_spot_lentigo"

Interstitial granulomatous dermatitis

Interstitial granulomatous dermatitis with arthritis is a condition that most commonly presents with symmetrical round-to-oval erythematous or violaceous plaques on the flanks, axillae, inner thighs, and lower abdomen.

Source (edited): "http://en.wikipedia.org/wiki/Interstitial_granulomatous_dermatitis"

Interstitial granulomatous drug reaction

Interstitial granulomatous drug reaction is an uncommon, yet under-recognized, pattern of adverse reactions to medication.

Source (edited): "http://en.wikipedia.org/wiki/Interstitial_granulomatous_drug_reaction"

Intraepidermal neutrophilic IgA dermatosis

Intraepidermal neutrophilic IgA dermatosis is characterized histologically by intraepidermal bullae with neutrophils, some eosinophils, and acantholysis.

Source (edited): "http://en.wikipedia.org/wiki/Intraepidermal_neutrophilic_IgA_dermatosis"

Intravascular large B-cell lymphoma

Intravascular large B-cell lymphoma, abbreviated **ILBCL** and also referred to as **angiotropic large-cell lymphoma**, **intralymphatic lymphomatosis**, **intravascular lymphomatosis**,, and, less specifically **intravascular lymphoma**.

Diagnosis

ILBCL is a condition that may present with non-specific symptoms and, thus, may be difficult to diagnose in a timely manner.

Presentations may include non-specific cutaneous lesions, and/or CNS involvement.

The diagnosis is established by the examination of tissue under the microscope (i.e. biopsy or autopsy) and immunohistochemical stains.

History

It used to be known as *malignant angioendotheliomatosis*, as it was once thought to arise from the endothelium.

Source (edited): "http://en.wikipedia.org/wiki/Intravascular_large_B-cell_lymphoma"

Intravascular lymphoma

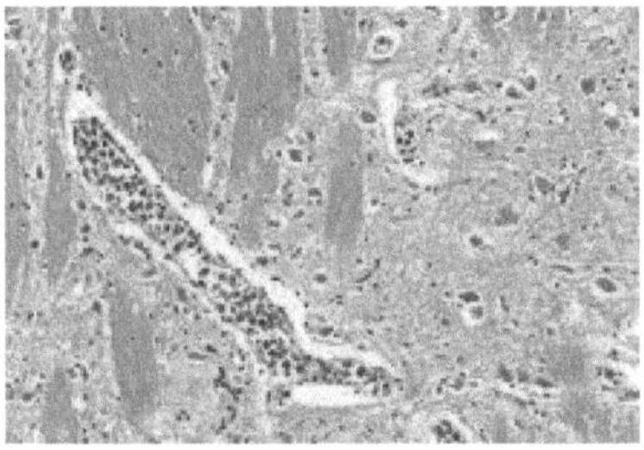

Micrograph showing an intravascular lymphoma in a blood vessel of the brain. H&E stain.

Intravascular lymphoma, also referred to as **angiotropic large cell lymphoma**,, **intralymphatic lymphomatosis**, **intravascular lymphomatosis**,, and "Malignant angioendotheliomatosis", is a condition that may present with variable symptoms, including various cutaneous morphologies (that are often very subtle and non-specific), and CNS symptoms.

Most intravascular lymphomas are of the B-cell lineage.

Diagnosis

ILBCL is a condition that may present with non-specific symptoms and, thus, may be difficult to diagnose in a timely manner.

Presentations may include non-specific cutaneous lesions, and/or CNS involvement.

The diagnosis is established by the examination of tissue under the microscope (i.e. biopsy or autopsy). Intravascular lymphomas have a large cell morphology, i.e. the malignant cells are two or more times the size of a normal lymphocyte, and typically have a prominent nucleolus.

Classification

- Intravascular large B-cell lymphoma
- Intravascular anaplastic large cell lymphoma

History

It used to be known as *malignant angioendotheliomatosis*, as it was once thought to arise from the endothelium.

Source (edited): "http://en.wikipedia.org/wiki/Intravascular_lymphoma"

Inverse psoriasis

Inverse psoriasis is a form of psoriasis that selectively and often exclusively involves the folds, recesses, and flexor surfaces such as the ears, axillae, groins, inframammary folds, navel, intergluteal crease, penis, lips, and webspaces.

Source (edited): "http://en.wikipedia.org/wiki/Inverse_psoriasis"

Iododerma

Iododermas are caused by iodides, with the most common sources of exposure being oral and intravenous contrast materials used to treat thyroid disease. The most common type of eruption is an acneiform eruption with numerous acutely inflamed follicular pustules, each surrounded by a ring of hyperemia.

Source (edited): "http://en.wikipedia.org/wiki/Iododerma"

Iron metallic discoloration

Iron metallic discoloration occurred more frequently in the past when soluble iron compounds were used in the treatment of allergic contact and other dermatitis, and in eroded areas iron was sometimes deposited in the skin, like a tattoo .

Source (edited): "http://en.wikipedia.org/wiki/Iron_metallic_discoloration"

Jadassohn–Pellizzari anetoderma

Jadassohn–Pellizzari anetoderma is a benign condition with focal loss of dermal elastic tissue. Anetodrma comes in three types: Primary anetoderma, secondary anetoderma, and familial anetoderma. Jadassohn-Pellizzari is one of two major classifications of primary anetoderma, the other being Schweninger–Buzzi anetoderma. The unlining difference between the two is that Jadassohn-Pellizzari anetoderma is preceded by inflammatory lesions.
Source (edited): "http://en.wikipedia.org/wiki/Jadassohn%E2%80%93Pellizzari_anetoderma"

Jaffe–Campanacci syndrome

Jaffe–Campanacci syndrome is one of the disorders associated with café au lait macules (CALMs). Presentations may include mental retardation, disseminated non-ossifying fibromas of the long bones and jaw, hypogonadism or cryptorchidism, or giant cell granulomas of the jaw.

It was characterized in 1958 and 1983.
Source (edited): "http://en.wikipedia.org/wiki/Jaffe%E2%80%93Campanacci_syndrome"

Janus kinase 3 deficiency

Janus kinase 3 deficiency or **JAK3 deficiency** is a defect in the body's cytokine receptors and their signaling. JAK3 encodes Janus kinase 3, a tyrosine kinase that belongs to the Janus family. JAK3 functions in signal transduction and interacts with members of the STAT (signal transduction and activators of transcription) family. The cause of JAK3 deficiency. The deficiency causes the near absence of T lymphocytes and Natural killer cells; and normal or elevated B lymphocytes due to an autosomal recessive variant of severe combined immunodeficiency (SCID)
Source (edited): "http://en.wikipedia.org/wiki/Janus_kinase_3_deficiency"

Jessner lymphocytic infiltrate of the skin

Jessner lymphocytic infiltrate of the skin (also known as "Benign lymphocytic infiltration of the skin," "Jessner lymphocytic infiltration of the skin," "Jessner–Kanof lymphocytic infiltration of the skin," and "Lymphocytic infiltrate of Jessner") is a cutaneous condition characterized by a persistent papular and plaque-like skin eruption. Thought to occur on the neck, face and back and may re-occur. This is a uncommon skin disease and is a benign collection of lymph cells. The cause of this is not known and can be hereditary.

It is named for Max Jessner.

It has been suggested that it is equivalent to lupus erythematosus tumidus.
Source (edited): "http://en.wikipedia.org/wiki/Jessner_lymphocytic_infiltrate_of_the_skin"

Johnson–McMillin syndrome

Johnson–McMillin syndrome is a neuroectodermal syndrome that consist of conductive hearing loss and microtia.
Source (edited): "http://en.wikipedia.org/wiki/Johnson%E2%80%93McMillin_syndrome"

Junctional epidermolysis bullosa with pyloric atresia

Junctional epidermolysis bullosa with pyloric atresia is a rare autosomal recessive form of junctional epidermolysis bullosa that presents at birth with severe mucocutaneous fragility and gastric outlet obstruction.

It can be associated with *ITGB4* or *ITGA6*.
Source (edited): "http://en.wikipedia.org/wiki/Junctional_epidermolysis_bullosa_with_pyloric_atresia"

Kairo cancer

Kairo cancer is a cutaneous condition that may develop due to hydrocarbon-fueled heat exposure from coal-fired clothing warmers.
Source (edited): "http://en.wikipedia.org/wiki/Kairo_cancer"

Kang cancer

Kang cancer is a cutaneous condition that may develop due to hydrocarbon-fueled heat exposure from sleeping on coal-fire-heated bricks.

Source (edited): "http://en.wikipedia.org/wiki/Kang_cancer"

Kangri ulcer

Kangri ulcers are a cutaneous condition prevalent among the poorer classes of Kashmir, and a consequence of wearing warm embers.

Source (edited): "http://en.wikipedia.org/wiki/Kangri_ulcer"

Keratinizing metaplasia

Keratinizing metaplasia is a condition affecting the epithelial surfaces of the body. It is caused by a dietary deficiency of vitamin A, a fat-soluble vitamin that is most often found in fats, milk, and some leafy vegetables.

Source (edited): "http://en.wikipedia.org/wiki/Keratinizing_metaplasia"

Keratocyst

A **keratocyst** is a type of cutaneous cyst. They appear similar to epidermoid cysts; however, are not limited to a specified location on the body. Keratocyst are most often reported in persons with nevoid basal cell carcinoma syndrome.

Pathology

Keratocysts have a stratified squamous epithelial wall without sebaceous lobules.

Source (edited): "http://en.wikipedia.org/wiki/Keratocyst"

Keratoderma

Keratoderma is a hornlike skin condition.

Classification

The keratodermas are classified into the following subgroups:

Congenital

- Simple keratodermas
  - Diffuse palmoplantar keratodermas
    - Diffuse epidermolytic palmoplantar keratoderma
    - Diffuse nonepidermolytic palmoplantar keratoderma
    - mal de Meleda
  - Focal palmoplantar keratoderma
    - Striate palmoplantar keratoderma
  - Punctate palmoplantar keratoderma
    - Keratosis punctata palmaris et plantaris
    - Spiny keratoderma
    - Focal acral hyperkeratosis
- Complex keratodermas
  - Diffuse palmoplantar keratoderma
    - Erythrokeratodermia variabilis
    - Palmoplantar keratoderma of Sybert
    - Olmsted syndrome
    - Naegeli-Franceschetti-Jadassohn syndrome
  - Focal palmoplantar keratoderma
    - Papillon-Lefèvre syndrome
    - Pachyonychia congenita type I
    - Pachyonychia congenita type II
    - Focal palmoplantar keratoderma with oral mucosal hyperkeratosis
    - Camisa disease
  - Ectodermal dysplasias
    - Clouston's hidrotic ectodermal dysplasia
    - Acrokeratotic poikiloderma
    - Dermatopathic pigmentosa reticularis
  - Syndromic keratodermas
    - Vohwinkel syndrome
    - Palmoplantar keratoderma associated with esophageal cancer
    - Palmoplantar keratoderma and spastic paraplegia
    - Naxos disease
    - Striate palmoplantar keratoderma, woolly hair, and left ventricular dilated cardiomyopathy
    - Keratitis-ichthyosis-deafness syndrome
    - Corneodermatosseous syndrome
    - Huriez syndrome
    - Oculocutaneous tyrosinemia
    - Cardiofaciocutaneous syndrome
    - Schöpf-Schulz-Passarge syndrome

Acquired

- Acquired keratodermas
  - AIDS-associated keratoderma
  - Arsenical keratoses

- Calluses
- Climacteric keratoderma
- Clavi (Corns)
- Eczema
- Human papillomavirus
- Keratoderma blenorrhagicum
- Lichen planus
- Norwegian scabies
- Paraneoplastic keratoderma
- Psoriasis
- Reiter's syndrome
- Secondary syphilis
- Tinea pedis
- Sézary syndrome
- Tuberculosis verrucosa cutis
- Drug-induced keratoderma

Source (edited): "http://en.wikipedia.org/wiki/Keratoderma"

Keratoderma climactericum

Keratoderma climactericum, also known as "Climacteric keratoderma," "Haxthausen's disease," and "Acquired plantar keratoderma," is a skin condition characterized by hyperkeratosis of the palms and soles beginning at about the time time of menopause.
Source (edited): "http://en.wikipedia.org/wiki/Keratoderma_climactericum"

Keratolysis exfoliativa

Keratolysis exfoliativa, (also known as "Lamellar dyshidrosis,", "Recurrent focal palmar peeling," "Recurrent palmar peeling") is a harmless condition of the skin. Although this particular condition is asymptomatic, it is often misdiagnosed as chronic contact dermatitis or psoriasis. It is primarily located on the palms of the hands and soles of the feet. It is characterized by dry skin and superficial, air-filled blisters. These blisters can be peeled off very easily and will leave reddish, tender areas. The loss of this horny layer of the skin, which protects the underlying layers, leaves the skin more vulnerable to dryness and cracking of the skin.

Causes

Keratolysis exfoliativa normally appears during warm weather. Due to excessive sweating and friction, in for example athletic shoes, the skin can start to exfoliate. Other factors that can cause exfoliation are detergents and solvents. Another very common cause has been reported from salt water fishermen, who often suffer from these symptoms. It is not sure whether it is from the salt water or whether it is from some bacteria from fish.

Treatment

Normally, exfoliation halts is restricted to a particular area and normal skin will replace the exfoliated parts, so no treatment is needed. Since keratolysis exfoliativa is caused by friction, detergents, and solvents, these factors should be avoided. Creams, especially those with silicone and lactic acid are also helpful. In severe cases, photochemotherapy is an option.

Prognosis

In most cases exfoliation resolves spontaneously and no lasting damage is seen.
Source (edited): "http://en.wikipedia.org/wiki/Keratolysis_exfoliativa"

Keratosis lichenoides chronica

Keratosis lichenoides chronica (also known as "Nekam's disease") is a rare dermatosis characterized by violaceous papular and nodular lesions, often arranged in a linear or reticulate pattern on the dorsal hands and feet, extremities, and buttock.
Source (edited): "http://en.wikipedia.org/wiki/Keratosis_lichenoides_chronica"

Keratosis punctata of the palmar creases

Keratosis punctata of the palmar creases (also known as "Hyperkeratosis penetrans," "Hyperkeratosis punctata," "Keratodermia punctata," "Keratosis punctata," "Keratotic pits of the palmar creases," "Lenticular atrophia of the palmar creases," and "Punctate keratosis of the palmar creases") is a common skin disorder that occurs most often in black patients, with skin lesions that are 1 to 5mm depressions filled with a comedo-like keratinous plug.

Treatment with etretinate has been described.
Source (edited): "http://en.wikipedia.org/wiki/Keratosis_punctata_of_the_palmar_creases"

Keratosis punctata palmaris et plantaris

Keratosis punctata palmaris et plantaris (also known as "Autosomal-dominant hereditary punctate keratoderma associated with malignancy," "Buschke–Fischer–Brauer disease," "Davis Colley disease," "Keratoderma disseminatum palmaris et plantaris," "Keratosis papulosa," "Keratoderma punctatum," "Keratodermia punctata," "Keratoma hereditarium dissipatum palmare et plantare," "Palmar and plantar seed dermatoses," "Palmar keratoses," "Papulotranslucent acrokeratoderma," "Punctate keratoderma," "Punctate keratoses of the palms and soles," and "Maculosa disseminata") is a skin condition, an autosomal dominant palmoplantar keratoderma with variable penetrance, characterized clinically by multiple, tiny, punctate keratoses over the entire palmoplantar surfaces, beginning over the lateral edge of the digits.

It has been linked to 15q22-q24.
Source (edited): "http://en.wikipedia.org/wiki/Keratosis_punctata_palmaris_et_plantaris"

Large plaque parapsoriasis

Large plaque parapsoriasis (also known as "parapsoriasis en plaques") are skin lesions that may be included in the modern scheme of cutaneous conditions described as parapsoriasis. These lesions, called plaques, may be irregularly round-shaped to oval and are 10 cm (3.9 in) or larger in diameter. They can be very thin plaques that are symptomatic or mildly pruritic. Large-plaque parapsoriasis is a common associate of retiform parapsoriasis, can be accompanied by poikiloderma vasculare atrophicans, and can in rare occasions be a precursor to cutaneous T-cell lymphoma.
Source (edited): "http://en.wikipedia.org/wiki/Large_plaque_parapsoriasis"

Lennert lymphoma

Lennert lymphoma (also known as "Lymphoepitheliod lymphoma") is a systemic T-cell lymphoma that presents with cutaneous skin lesions roughly 10% of the time.
Source (edited): "http://en.wikipedia.org/wiki/Lennert_lymphoma"

Lentigo maligna melanoma

Lentigo maligna melanoma is a melanoma that has evolved from a lentigo maligna. They are usually found on chronically sun damaged skin such as the face and the forearms of the elderly. The nomenclature is very confusing to both patients and physicians alike.

Lentigo maligna is the non-invasive skin growth that some pathologists consider to be a melanoma-in-situ. A few pathologists do not consider lentigo maligna to be a melanoma at all, but a precursor to melanomas. Once a lentigo maligna becomes a lentigo maligna melanoma, it is treated as if it were an invasive melanoma.

Presentation

An invasive tumor arising from a classical lentigo maligna. Usually a darkly pigmented raised papule or nodule, arising from a patch of irregularly pigmented flat brown to dark brown lesion of sun exposed skin of the face or arms in an elderly patient.

Diagnosis

First dilemma in diagnosis is recognition. As lentigo malignas often present on severely sun damaged skin, it is frequently found amongst numerous pigmented lesions - thin seborrheic keratoses, lentigo senilis, lentigines. It is difficult to distinguish these lesions with the naked eye alone, and even with some difficulty using dermatoscopy. As the lentigo maligna is often very large, it often merges with, or encompasses other skin tumors - such as lentigines, melanocytic nevi, and seborrheic keratosis.

Second dilemma is the biopsy technique. Even though excisional biopsy (removing the entire lesion) is ideal, and advocated by pathologists; practical reason dictates that this should not be done. These tumors are often large and presenting on the facial area. Excision of such large tumor would be absolutely contraindicated if the lesion's identity is uncertain. The preferred method of diagnosis is by using a shave biopsy because punch biopsies give up to an 80% false negative rate. While one section of the tumor might show benign melanocytic nevus, another section might show features concerning of severe cellular atypia. When cellular atypia is noted, a pathologist might indicate that the entire lesion should be removed. It is at this point that one can comfortable remove the entire lesion, and thus confirming the final diagnosis of lentigo maligna. Despite the high false negative rate, ouch biopsies are often used and the size of the punch biopsy can vary from 1 mm to 2 mm, but it is preferred to use a punch 1.5 mm or larger. Representative samples of the most atypical part of the nevus should be biopsy, often by the aid of dermatoscopy.

Treatment

Is dependent on the thickness of the invasive component of the lentigo maligna. Treatment is essentially identical to other melanomas of the same thickness and stage.
Source (edited): "http://en.wikipedia.

org/wiki/Lentigo_maligna_melanoma"

Lentigo simplex

Lentigo simplex (also known as "Simple lentigo") is the most common form of lentigo. A single lesion or multiple lesions (lentigines) may be present at birth or more commonly first develop in early childhood. Lentigo simplex is not induced by sun exposure, and it is not associated with any medical diseases or conditions. It is also referred to as *simple lentigo* and *juvenile lentigo*.
Source (edited): "http://en.wikipedia.org/wiki/Lentigo_simplex"

Leukemia cutis

Leukemia cutis is the infiltration of neoplastic leukocytes or their precursors into the skin resulting in clinically identifiable cutaneous lesions. This condition may be contrasted with leukemids, which are skin lesions that occur with leukemia, but which are not related to leukemic cell infiltration. Leukemia cutis can occur in most forms of leukemia,including chronic myeloid leukemia, acute lymphoblastic leukemia, chronic lymphocytic leukemia, acute myeloid leukemia, and prolymphocytic leukemia.
Source (edited): "http://en.wikipedia.org/wiki/Leukemia_cutis"

Leukemid

Leukemids (also known as "Nonspecific cutaneous conditions associated with leukemia") are nonspecific skin lesions that occur with leukemia which are not related to leukemic cell infiltration. This condition may be contrasted with leukemia cutis, which is the infiltration of neoplastic leukocytes or their precursors into the skin resulting in clinically identifiable cutaneous lesions.
Source (edited): "http://en.wikipedia.org/wiki/Leukemid"

Leukocyte adhesion molecule deficiency

Leukocyte adhesion molecule deficiency is a rare autosomal recessive disorder characterized by recurrent bacterial and fungal infections and impaired neutrophil migration.
Source (edited): "http://en.wikipedia.org/wiki/Leukocyte_adhesion_molecule_deficiency"

Leukoderma

Leukoderma is a cutaneous condition, an acquired condition with localized loss of pigmentation of the skin that may occur after any number of inflammatory skin conditions, burns, intralesional steroid injections, postdermabrasion, etc.

Traditional Therapy

The bael fruit is traditionally used to treat this condition.
Source (edited): "http://en.wikipedia.org/wiki/Leukoderma"

Leukoplakia with tylosis and esophageal carcinoma

Leukoplakia with tylosis and esophageal carcinoma is a rare condition characterized by leukoplakia associated with esophageal carcinoma.
Source (edited): "http://en.wikipedia.org/wiki/Leukoplakia_with_tylosis_and_esophageal_carcinoma"

Leukotriene receptor antagonist-associated Churg–Strauss syndrome

Leukotriene receptor antagonist-associated Churg–Strauss syndrome may occur in asthma patients being treated with leukotriene receptor antagonists, occurring 2 days to 10 months after the antagonist has been started,

with features of the syndrome including peripheral eosinphilia, pulmonary infiltrates, and less commonly neuropathy, sinusitis, and cardiomyopathy.
Source (edited): "http://en.wikipedia.org/wiki/Leukotriene_receptor_antagonist-associated_Churg%E2%80%93Strauss_syndrome"

Lichen amyloidosis

Lichen amyloidosis is a cutaneous condition characterized by the appearance of occasionally itchy lichenoid papules, typically appearing bilaterally on the shins.
Source (edited): "http://en.wikipedia.org/wiki/Lichen_amyloidosis"

Lichen aureus

Lichen aureus (also known as "lichen purpuricus") is a skin condition characterized by the sudden appearance of one or several golden or rust-colored, closely packed macules or lichenoid papules.
Source (edited): "http://en.wikipedia.org/wiki/Lichen_aureus"

Lichen planus actinicus

Lichen planus actinicus (also known as "Actinic lichen niditus," "Actinic lichen planus," "Lichen planus atrophicus annularis," "Lichen planus subtropicus," "Lichen planus tropicus," "Lichenoid melanodermatitis," "Lichenoid melanodermatosis," and "Summertime actinic lichenoid eruption") is a variant of lichen planus that is more common in Middle Eastern countries in spring and summer, where sunlight appears to have a precipitating effect, such that exposed areas of the face, dorsal hands and arms, and nape of the neck are usually affected by papules that are hyperpigmented and violaceous-brown in color with a thready, rolled edge showing well-defined borders.
Source (edited): "http://en.wikipedia.org/wiki/Lichen_planus_actinicus"

Lichen planus pemphigoides

Lichen planus pemphigoides is characterized by the development of tense blisters atop lesions of lichen planus or the development vesicles de novo on uninvolved skin. It is important to differentiate this entity from bullous lichen planus, in which blisters develop in skin lesions of longstanding lichen planus as a result of intense lichenoid inflammation and extensive liquefaction degeneration of basal keratinocytes.
Source (edited): "http://en.wikipedia.org/wiki/Lichen_planus_pemphigoides"

Lichen planus pigmentosus

Lichen planus pigmentosus is an uncommon variant of lichen planus characterized by hyperpigmented, dark-brown macules in sun-exposed areas and flexural folds.
Source (edited): "http://en.wikipedia.org/wiki/Lichen_planus_pigmentosus"

Lichen planus–lichen sclerosus overlap syndrome

Lichen planus–lichen sclerosus overlap syndrome is a rare skin condition characterized by skin lesions of lichen planus and lichen sclerosus.
Source (edited): "http://en.wikipedia.org/wiki/Lichen_planus%E2%80%93lichen_sclerosus_overlap_syndrome"

Lichen striatus

Lichen striatus (also known as "Blaschko linear acquired inflammatory skin eruption" and "Linear lichenoid dermatosis") is a rare skin condition that is seen primarily in children, most frequently appearing ages 5-15.
Source (edited): "http://en.wikipedia.org/wiki/Lichen_striatus"

Lichenoid dermatitis

Lichenoid dermatitis represents a wide range of cutaneous disorders characterized by lichen planus-like skin lesions.
Source (edited): "http://en.wikipedia.org/wiki/Lichenoid_dermatitis"

Lichenoid keratosis

Lichenoid keratoses (also known as "Benign lichenoid keratosis," "Lichen planus-like keratosis," "Solitary lichenoid keratosis," and "Solitary lichen planus") are a cutaneous condition characterized by brown to red, scaling maculopapules found on sun-exposed skin of extremities. Restated, this is a cutaneous condition usually characterized by a solitary dusky-red to violaceous papular skin lesion.
Source (edited): "http://en.wikipedia.org/wiki/Lichenoid_keratosis"

Lichenoid reaction of graft-versus-host disease

Lichenoid reaction of graft-versus-host disease presents with chronic graft-versus-host disease, characterized by a lichenoid eruption indistinguishable clinically and histologically from lichen planus.
Source (edited): "http://en.wikipedia.org/wiki/Lichenoid_reaction_of_graft-versus-host_disease"

Linear IgA bullous dermatosis

Linear IgA bullous dermatosis (also known as "Linear IgA dermatosis") is frequently associated with medication exposure, especially vancomycin, with men and women being equally affected.
Linear IgA dermatosis is a rare immune-mediated blistering skin disease that may be divided into two types, chronic bullous disease of childhood and adult linear IgA disease.
Source (edited): "http://en.wikipedia.org/wiki/Linear_IgA_bullous_dermatosis"

Linear focal elastosis

Linear focal elastosis (also known as "Elastotic striae") presents with asymptomatic, palpable or atrophic, yellow lines of the middle and lower back, thighs, arms and breasts.
Source (edited): "http://en.wikipedia.org/wiki/Linear_focal_elastosis"

Linear lichen planus

Linear lichen planus may develop secondary to trauma (koebnerization) or, uncommonly, as a spontaneous, isolated eruption, usually on the extremities, and rarely on the face.
Source (edited): "http://en.wikipedia.org/wiki/Linear_lichen_planus"

Linear scleroderma

Linear scleroderma is a type of localized scleroderma which is an auto-immune disorder characterized by a line of thickened skin which can affect the bones and muscles underneath it.

Presentation

It most often occurs in the arms, legs, or forehead, and may occur in more than one area.

It is also most likely to be on just one side of the body.

Linear scleroderma generally first appears in young children.
Source (edited): "http://en.wikipedia.org/wiki/Linear_scleroderma"

Lipoatrophia annularis

Lipoatrophia annularis (also known as "Ferreira–Marques lipoatrophia") is a skin condition affecting primarily

women, characterized by the loss of subcutaneous fat in the upper extremity. It is a form of lipodystrophy.
Source (edited): "http://en.wikipedia.org/wiki/Lipoatrophia_annularis"

Livedoid dermatitis

Livedoid dermatitis (also known as "Embolia cutis medicamentosa," and "Nicolau syndrome") occurs immediately after an intramuscular injection, and is characterized by intense pain and blanching of the overlying skin, known as ischemic pallor.
Source (edited): "http://en.wikipedia.org/wiki/Livedoid_dermatitis"

Localized granuloma annulare

Localized granuloma annulare is a skin condition of unknown cause, tending to affect children and young to middle-aged adults, usually appearing on the lateral or dorsal surfaces of the fingers or hands, elbows, dorsal feet, and ankles.
Source (edited): "http://en.wikipedia.org/wiki/Localized_granuloma_annulare"

Localized lichen myxedematosus

Localized lichen myxedematosus is a group of skin condition caused by fibroblasts producing abnormally large amounts of mucopolysaccharides, a disease for which there is no treatment.
Source (edited): "http://en.wikipedia.org/wiki/Localized_lichen_myxedematosus"

Localized lipodystrophy

Localized lipodystrophy is a skin condition characterized by the loss subcutaneous fat localized to sites of insulin injection.
Source (edited): "http://en.wikipedia.org/wiki/Localized_lipodystrophy"

Localized morphea

Localized morphea is a form of scleroderma that is twice as common in women as in men, occurs in childhood as well as in adult life, and most often presents as macules or plaques a few centimeters in diameter, but also may occur as bands or in guttate lesions or nodules.
Source (edited): "http://en.wikipedia.org/wiki/Localized_morphea"

Localized pustular psoriasis

Localized pustular psoriasis presents as two distinct conditions that must be considered separate from generalized psoriasis, and without systemic symptoms, these two distinct varieties being pustulosis palmaris et plantaris and acrodermatitis continua.
Source (edited): "http://en.wikipedia.org/wiki/Localized_pustular_psoriasis"

Lupoid rosacea

Lupoid rosacea (also known as "Granulomatous rosacea," "Micropapular tuberculid", or "Rosacea-like tuberculid of Lewandowsky") is characterized by the development of epithelioid (lupoid) granulomas in a diffuse pattern.
Source (edited): "http://en.wikipedia.org/wiki/Lupoid_rosacea"

Lupus erythematosus

Lupus erythematosus is a category for a collection of diseases with similar underlying problems with immunity (autoimmune disease). Symptoms of these diseases can affect many different body systems, including joints, skin, kidneys, blood cells, heart, and lungs. Four main types of lupus exist — systemic lupus erythematosus, discoid lupus erythematosus, drug-induced lupus erythematosus, and neonatal lupus erythematosus. Of these, systemic lupus erythematosus is the most common and serious form of lupus.

Photosensitivity's relationship to and influence on the systemic manifestations of lupus remain to be defined. Mechanisms for photosensitivity might include: modulation of autoantibody location, cytotoxic effects, apoptosis induction with autoantigens in apoptotic blebs, upregulation of adhesion molecules and cytokines, induction of nitric oxide synthase expression and ultraviolet-generated antigenic DNA. Tumor necrosis factor alpha also seems to play a role in the development of photosensitivity.

Types

Lupus erythematosus may manifest as a systemic disease or in purely cutaneous forms. Types of lupus erythematous can be categorized into the following types:

- Acute cutaneous lupus erythematosus
- Subacute cutaneous lupus erythematosus
- Chronic cutaneous lupus erythematosus
  - Discoid lupus erythematosus
    - Childhood discoid lupus erythematosus
    - Generalized discoid lupus erythematosus
    - Localized discoid lupus erythematosus
  - Chilblain lupus erythematosus (Hutchinson)
  - Lupus erythematosus-lichen planus overlap syndrome
  - Lupus erythematosus panniculitis (Lupus erythematosus profundus)
  - Tumid lupus erythematosus
  - Verrucous lupus erythematosus (Hypertrophic lupus erythematosus)
- Complement deficiency syndromes
- Drug-induced lupus erythematosus
- Neonatal lupus erythematosus
- Systemic lupus erythematosus

Source (edited): "http://en.wikipedia.org/wiki/Lupus_erythematosus"

Lupus erythematosus panniculitis

Lupus erythematosus panniculitis (also known as "Lupus erythematosus profundus," "Lupus panniculitis," "Lupus profundus", and "Subcutaneous lupus erythematosus") presents with subcutaneous nodules that are commonly firm, sharply defined, and nontender.
Source (edited): "http://en.wikipedia.org/wiki/Lupus_erythematosus_panniculitis"

Lupus erythematosus–lichen planus overlap syndrome

Lupus erythematosus–lichen planus overlap syndrome (also known as "Lichen planus–lupus erythematosus overlap syndrome") is a true overlap syndrome with features of both lupus erythematosus and lichen planus, with skin lesions usually large, atropic, hypopigmented, red or pink patches and plaques.

Lichen planus–lupus erythematosus overlap syndrome is a rare variant of lichen planus characterized by lesions that share features with lupus erythematosus. Atrophic plaques and patches with hypopigmentation and a livid red to blue-violet color with telangiectasia and minimal scaling are characteristic.
Source (edited): "http://en.wikipedia.org/wiki/Lupus_erythematosus%E2%80%93lichen_planus_overlap_syndrome"

Lupus miliaris disseminatus faciei

Lupus miliaris disseminatus faciei is a disease with a similar appearance to acne vulgaris.
Source (edited): "http://en.wikipedia.org/wiki/Lupus_miliaris_disseminatus_faciei"

Lupus pernio

Lupus pernio is a chronic raised indurated (hardened) lesion of the skin, often purplish in color. It resembles frostbite as it is seen on ears, cheeks, lips, nose, hands, fingers and forehead. It is most often associated with sarcoidosis. Microscopically, it resembles lupus vulgaris. Biopsy shows granulomatous infiltration.
Source (edited): "http://en.wikipedia.org/wiki/Lupus_pernio"

Lycopenemia

Lycopenemia is a skin condition caused by excessive ingestion of red foods, such as tomatoes, beets, chili beans, and various fruits and berries, which leads to a reddish discoloration of the skin.

Source (edited): "http://en.wikipedia.org/wiki/Lycopenemia"

Lymphedema praecox

Lymphedema praecox is a condition characterized by swelling of the soft tissues in which an excessive amount of lymph has accumulated, and generally develops in females between the ages of nine and twenty-five.

Source (edited): "http://en.wikipedia.org/wiki/Lymphedema_praecox"

Lymphedema–distichiasis syndrome

Lymphedema–distichiasis syndrome is a medical condition associated with the FOXC2 gene.

Source (edited): "http://en.wikipedia.org/wiki/Lymphedema%E2%80%93distichiasis_syndrome"

Macular amyloidosis

Macular amyloidosis, located on the right lumbar region of the back

Macular amyloidosis is a cutaneous condition characterized by itchy, brown, rippled macules usually located on the interscapular region of the back.

Source (edited): "http://en.wikipedia.org/wiki/Macular_amyloidosis"

Majocchi's disease

Majocchi's disease (also known as "Purpura annularis telangiectodes," and "Purpura annularis telangiectodes of Majocchi") is a skin condition characterized by bluish-red 1- to 3-cm annular patches composed of dark red telangiectases with petechiae.

Source (edited): "http://en.wikipedia.org/wiki/Majocchi%27s_disease"

Major aphthous ulcer

Major aphthous ulcer (also known as "Periadenitis mucosa necrotica recurrens") is a condition of the oral mucosa characterized by a painful, shotlike nodule on the inner lip, buccal mucosa, or tongue.

Source (edited): "http://en.wikipedia.org/wiki/Major_aphthous_ulcer"

Malignant blue nevus

A **malignant blue nevus** is a cutaneous condition characterized by a sheet-like growth pattern, mitoses, necrosis, and cellular atypia.

Source (edited): "http://en.wikipedia.org/wiki/Malignant_blue_nevus"

Malum perforans pedis

Malum perforans pedis (also known as a "Neurotrophic ulcer," and "Perforating ulcer of the foot") is a cutaneous condition of chronic, trophic, ulcerative disease seen on the sole in denervating diseases, particularly tabes dorsalis.

Source (edited): "http://en.wikipedia.org/wiki/Malum_perforans_pedis"

Marshall–White syndrome

Marshall–White syndrome is a skin condition that consists of Bier spots associated with insomnia and tachycardia.

Source (edited): "http://en.wikipedia.org/wiki/Marshall%E2%80%93White_syndrome"

Median rhomboid glossitis

Median rhomboid glossitis (also known as "Central papillary atrophy") is a condition characterized by a shiny oval or diamond-shaped elevation, invariably situated on the dorsum of the tongue in the midline immediately in front of the circumvallate papillae.

Source (edited): "http://en.wikipedia.org/wiki/Median_rhomboid_glossitis"

Medication-induced hyperlipoproteinemia

Medication-induced hyperlipoproteinemia is a condition that results from the decreasing of lipoprotein lipase activity resulting in eruptive xanthomas.

Source (edited): "http://en.wikipedia.org/wiki/Medication-induced_hyperlipoproteinemia"

Medium-sized congenital nevocytic nevus

Medium-sized congenital nevocytic nevus is a cutaneous condition characterized by a nevus, generally defined as having a diameter more than 2cm but less than 20cm.

Source (edited): "http://en.wikipedia.org/wiki/Medium-sized_congenital_nevocytic_nevus"

Melanocytic oral lesion

Melanocytic oral lesions are an extremely uncommon condition characterized by pigmented lesions of the mucous membranes.

Source (edited): "http://en.wikipedia.org/wiki/Melanocytic_oral_lesion"

Mercury granuloma

Mercury granulomas is the result of mercury exposure, a skin condition characterized by foreign-body giant cell reaction.

Source (edited): "http://en.wikipedia.org/wiki/Mercury_granuloma"

Metastatic calcinosis cutis

Metastatic calcinosis cutis is a cutaneous condition characterized by calcification of the skin resulting from the deposition of calcium and phosphorus, and associated with an internal malignancy.

Source (edited): "http://en.wikipedia.org/wiki/Metastatic_calcinosis_cutis"

Methotrexate-induced papular eruption

Methotrexate-induced papular eruption appears in patients being treated with methotrexate, such as those with rheumatic disease, presenting with erythematous indurated papules, usually located on the proximal extremities.

It has been suggested that it may represent a Cutaneous small-vessel vasculitis.

Source (edited): "http://en.wikipedia.org/wiki/Methotrexate-induced_papular_eruption"

Metophyma

Metophyma refers to cushion-like swellings on the forehead above the saddle of the nose.

Source (edited): "http://en.wikipedia.org/wiki/Metophyma"

Microscopic polyangiitis

Microscopic polyangiitis (also known as "Microscopic polyarteritis," "Microscopic polyarteritis nodosa," "MPA") is an ill-defined autoimmune disease characterized by pauci-immune, necrotizing, small-vessel vasculitis without clinical or pathological evidence of necrotizing granulomatous inflammation.

Presentation

Because many different organ systems may be involved, a wide range of symptoms are possible in MPA.

Purpura and livedo may be present.

Diagnosis

Laboratory tests show an increased sedimentation rate, reduced red blood count, antineutrophil cytoplasmic antibodies (p-ANCA) directed against myeloperoxidase (a constituent of neutrophil granules), and protein and red blood cells in the urine.

The test for anti-glomerular basement membrane antibody (GBM), which is positive in Goodpasture's syndrome, is negative.

Cause

This condition, the clinical picture of which may include many features of systemic lupus erythematosis, has been reported. While the mechanism of disease has yet to be fully elucidated, the leading hypothesis is that the process is begun with an autoimmune process of unknown etiology that triggers production of p-ANCA. These antibodies will circulate at low levels until a pro-inflammatory trigger - such as infection, malignancy, or drug therapy. The trigger upregulates production of p-ANCA. Then, the large number of antibodies make it more likely that they will bind a neutrophil. Once bound, the neutrophil degranulates. The degranulation releases toxins that cause endothelial injury, that is, damage to vessels of glomeruli.

Treatment

The customary treatment involves long term dosage of prednisone, alternated or combined with cytotoxic drugs, such as cyclophosphamide or azathioprine.

Plasmapheresis may also be indicated in the acute setting to remove ANCA antibodies.

Rituximab has been investigated, and in April 2011 approved by the FDA when used in combination with glucocorticoids.

Source (edited): "http://en.wikipedia.org/wiki/Microscopic_polyangiitis"

Miliaria crystallina

Miliaria crystalline (also known as "Miliaria crystallina," and "Sudamina") is a skin condition characterized by small, clear, and very superficial vesicles with no inflammatory reaction.

Source (edited): "http://en.wikipedia.org/wiki/Miliaria_crystallina"

Miliaria profunda

Miliaria profunda (also known as "Mammillaria") is a skin condition characterized by non-pruritic, flesh-colored, deep-seated, whitish papules.

Source (edited): "http://en.wikipedia.org/wiki/Miliaria_profunda"

Miliaria pustulosa

Miliaria pustulosa is a skin condition, a type of miliaria, that is preceded by another dermatitis that has produced injury, destruction, or blocking of the sweat duct.

Source (edited): "http://en.wikipedia.org/wiki/Miliaria_pustulosa"

Molluscum dermatitis

Molluscum dermatitis represents a unique form of id reaction, in which patients may present with localized or widespread eczema surrounding scattered lesions of molluscum contagiosum.

Source (edited): "http://en.wikipedia.org/wiki/Molluscum_dermatitis"

Mondor's disease

Mondor's disease (also known as "Mondor's syndrome of superficial thrombophlebitis") is a rare condition which involves thrombophlebitis of the superficial veins of the breast and anterior chest wall. It sometimes occurs in the arm or penis.

Patients with this disease often have abrupt onset of superficial pain, with possible swelling and redness of a limited area of their anterior chest wall or breast. There is usually a lump present, which may be somewhat linear and tender. Because of the possibility of the lump being from another cause, patients are often referred for mammogram and/or breast ultrasound.

Mondor's disease is self limiting and generally benign. A cause is often not identified, but when found include trauma, surgery, or inflammation such as infection. There have been occasional cases of associated malignancy. Management is with warm compresses and pain relievers, most commonly NSAIDS such as ibuprofen.

It is named after Henri Mondor (1885-1962), a surgeon in Paris, France who first described the disease in 1939.

Source (edited): "http://en.wikipedia.org/wiki/Mondor%27s_disease"

Morphea profunda

Morphea profunda involves deep subcutaneous tissue, including fascia, and there is a clinical overlap with eosinophilic fasciitis, eosinophilia-myalgia syndrome, and the Spanish toxic oil syndrome. Morphea profunda shows little response to corticosteroids and tends to run a more chronic debilitating course.

Source (edited): "http://en.wikipedia.org/wiki/Morphea_profunda"

Morpheaform sarcoidosis

Morpheaform sarcoidosis is a very rare cutaneous condition characterized by specific cutaneous skin lesions of sarcoidosis accompanied by substantial fibrosis, simulating morphea.

Source (edited): "http://en.wikipedia.org/wiki/Morpheaform_sarcoidosis"

Morphea–lichen sclerosus et atrophicus overlap

Morphea–lichen sclerosus et atrophicus overlap is characterized by both lesions of morphea and lichen sclerosus et atrophicus, most commonly seen in women.

Source (edited): "http://en.wikipedia.org/wiki/Morphea%E2%80%93lichen_sclerosus_et_atrophicus_overlap"

Moynahan syndrome

Moynahan syndrome is a cutaneous condition characterized by multiple lentigines, congenital mitral stenosis, dwarfism, genital hypoplasia, and mental deficiency.

It was characterized in 1962.

It is one of three conditions named for Edmund John Moynahan.

Source (edited): "http://en.wikipedia.org/wiki/Moynahan_syndrome"

Mucinosis

Mucinoses are a group of cutaneous diseases caused by fibroblasts producing abnormally large amounts of acid mucopolysaccharides (i.e. mucin), usually hyaluronic acid.

Source (edited): "http://en.wikipedia.org/wiki/Mucinosis"

Mucosal lentigines

Mucosal lentigines (also known as "Labial, penile, and vulvar melanosis," and "Melanotic macules") is a cutaneous condition characterized by light brown macules on mucosal surfaces.
Source (edited): "http://en.wikipedia.org/wiki/Mucosal_lentigines"

Mucosal melanoma

Mucosal melanoma is a rare cutaneous condition characterized by a melanoma of the mucous membranes.
Source (edited): "http://en.wikipedia.org/wiki/Mucosal_melanoma"

Mucosal sarcoidosis

Mucosal sarcoidosis is a cutaneous condition characterized by pinhead-sized papules that may be grouped and fused together to form a flat plaque.
Source (edited): "http://en.wikipedia.org/wiki/Mucosal_sarcoidosis"

Multicentric reticulohistiocytosis

Multicentric reticulohistiocytosis is a multisystem disease beginning usually around the age of 50 years old, and is twice as common in women.
Source (edited): "http://en.wikipedia.org/wiki/Multicentric_reticulohistiocytosis"

Napkin psoriasis

Napkin psoriasis, or psoriasis in the diaper area, is characteristically seen in infants between two and eight months of age.
Source (edited): "http://en.wikipedia.org/wiki/Napkin_psoriasis"

Narcotic dermopathy

Narcotic dermopathy is a skin condition caused by the injection of drugs intravenously, resulting in thrombosed, cordlike, thickened veins at the site of injection.
Source (edited): "http://en.wikipedia.org/wiki/Narcotic_dermopathy"

Necrobiosis lipoidica

Necrobiosis lipoidica is a necrotizing skin condition that usually occurs in patients with diabetes but can also be associated with Rheumatoid Arthritis. In such cases it may be called **necrobiosis lipoidica diabeticorum (NLD)**. NLD occurs in approximately 0.3% of the diabetic population, with the majority of sufferers being women (approximately 90%).

Necrobiosis lipoidica is closely related to granuloma annulare.

Clinical appearance

NL/NLD most frequently appears on the patient's shins, often on both legs. The lesions are often tender and may become yellowish in the centre and ulcerate when injured. The first symptom of NL/NLD is often a "bruised" appearance (erythematous) that is not necessarily associated with a known injury. The extent to which NL/NLD is inherited is not known.
Source (edited): "http://en.wikipedia.org/wiki/Necrobiosis_lipoidica"

Necrobiotic xanthogranuloma

Necrobiotic xanthogranuloma (also known as "Necrobiotic xanthogranuloma with paraproteinemia") is a multisystem disease that affects older adults, and is characterized by prominent skin findings.
Source (edited): "http://en.wikipedia.org/wiki/Necrobiotic_xanthogranuloma"

Neonatal acne

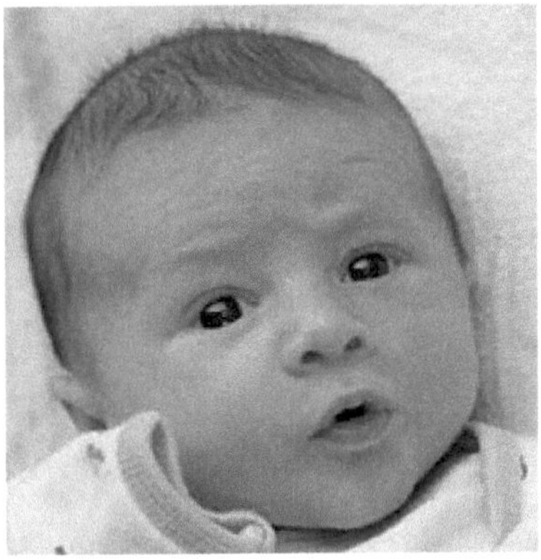

An infant with neotanal acne on the face, especially the forehead

Neonatal acne (also known as "Acne infantum," "Acne neonatorum", and "Neonatal cephalic pustulosis") is an acneiform eruption that occurs in newborns or infants, and is often seen on the nose and adjacent portions of the cheeks..

The main cause of this condition is not known, but it could be due to the increased sensitivity of the infant's sebaceous glands to maternal hormones during pregnancy which also leads to a variety of skin conditions in the newborn.Typically, it peaks at around 2 months and rarely needs treatment. Sometimes gels or ointments are given.

Source (edited): "http://en.wikipedia.org/wiki/Neonatal_acne"

Neonatal lupus erythematosus

Neonatal lupus erythematosus is the occurrence of SLE symptoms in an infant born from a mother with SLE, most commonly presenting with a rash resembling discoid lupus erythematosus, and sometimes with systemic abnormalities such as heart block or hepatosplenomegaly.

The infants have no skin lesions at birth, but develop them during the first weeks of life. Neonatal lupus is usually benign and self-limited.

It is associated with mothers who carry the Ro/SSA antibody.

Source (edited): "http://en.wikipedia.org/wiki/Neonatal_lupus_erythematosus"

Neuropathic ulcer

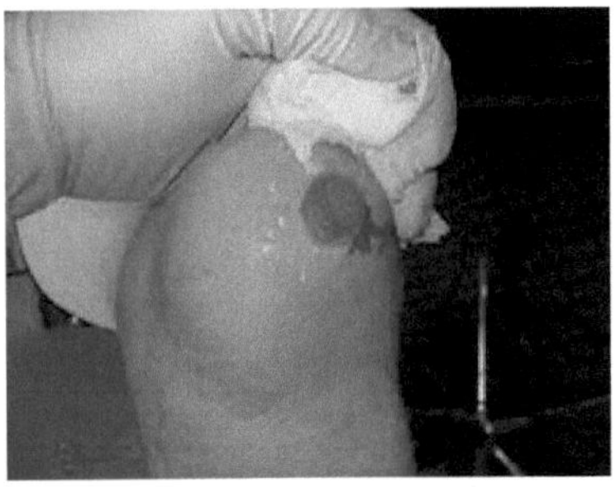

Neuropathic ulcer of the heel, a very common location

Neuropathic ulcers (also known as "Mal perforans") are skin lesions that are common in diabetics. They are usually related to sensory loss in the lower extremities.

Source (edited): "http://en.wikipedia.org/wiki/Neuropathic_ulcer"

Neurotic excoriations

Neurotic excoriations is a condition in which patients produce skin lesions through repetitive, compulsive excoriation of their skin.

Source (edited): "http://en.wikipedia.org/wiki/Neurotic_excoriations"

Neutrophilic dermatosis of the dorsal hands

Neutrophilic dermatosis of the dorsal hands (also known as "Pustular vasculitis of the dorsal hands") is a skin condition that presents with edematous pustular or ulcerative nodules or plaques localized to the dorsal hands.
Source (edited): "http://en.wikipedia.org/wiki/Neutrophilic_dermatosis_of_the_dorsal_hands"

Nevus of Ito

Nevus of Ito (also known as "Nevus fuscoceruleus acromiodeltoideus") is a cutaneous condition with similar features to the Nevus of Ota, but occurring in a different distribution.
Source (edited): "http://en.wikipedia.org/wiki/Nevus_of_Ito"

Nevus spilus

Nevus spilus (also known as **speckled lentiginous nevus** and **zosteriform lentiginous nevus**) is a skin lesion that presents as a light brown or tan macule, speckled with smaller, darker macules or papules.
Source (edited): "http://en.wikipedia.org/wiki/Nevus_spilus"

Nodular amyloidosis

Nodular amyloidosis is a rare cutaneous condition characterized by nodules that involve the acral areas.
Source (edited): "http://en.wikipedia.org/wiki/Nodular_amyloidosis"

Nodular vasculitis

Nodular vasculitis is a skin condition characterized by crops of small, tender, erythematous nodules on the legs, mostly on the calves and shins. Miroscopically there are epithelioid granulomas and vasculitis in the subcutaneous tissue, making it a form of panicullitis. Most of these cases are now thought to be manifestation of tuberculosis and indeed they respond well to anti-tuberculous treatment.
Source (edited): "http://en.wikipedia.org/wiki/Nodular_vasculitis"

Non-X histiocytosis

Non-X histiocytoses are a clinically well-defined group of cutaneous syndromes characterized by infiltrates of monocytes/macrophages, as opposed to X-type histiocytoses in which the infiltrates contain Langerhans cells. Conditions included in this group are:

- Juvenile xanthogranuloma
- Benign cephalic histiocytosis
- Generalized eruptive histiocytoma
- Xanthoma disseminatum
- Progressive nodular histiocytosis
- Papular xanthoma
- Hereditary progressive mucinous histiocytosis
- Reticulohistiocytosis
- Indeterminate cell histiocytosis
- Sea-blue histiocytosis

Source (edited): "http://en.wikipedia.org/wiki/Non-X_histiocytosis"

Non-mycosis fungoides CD30− cutaneous large T-cell lymphoma

Non-mycosis fungoides CD30− cutaneous large T-cell lymphoma is a cutaneous condition that usually presents as solitary or generalized plaques, nodules, or tumors of short duration.
Source (edited): "http://en.wikipedia.org/wiki/Non-mycosis_fungoides_CD30%E2%88%92_cutaneous_large_T-cell_lymphoma"

Normolipoproteinemic xanthomatosis

Normolipoproteinemic xanthomatosis is a cutaneous condition characterized by a xanthoma in the presence of

normal cholesterol and lipoprotein levels.
Source (edited): "http://en.wikipedia.org/wiki/Normolipoproteinemic_xanthomatosis"

Nutritional deficiency eczema

Nutritional deficiency eczema is a pattern of eczema with localized, thickened, scaling patches that have some characteristics of nummular eczema, seborrheic dermatitis, and neurodermatitis that may be seen in alcoholics.
Source (edited): "http://en.wikipedia.org/wiki/Nutritional_deficiency_eczema"

Obstructive purpura

Obstructive purpura is a skin condition that may result from mechanical obstruction to circulation, with resulting stress on the small vessels leading to purpura.
Source (edited): "http://en.wikipedia.org/wiki/Obstructive_purpura"

Occlusion miliaria

Occlusion miliaria is a skin condition that is accompanied by anhidrosis and increased heat-stress susceptibility, all after the application of extensive polyethylene film occlusion for 48 hours or longer.
Source (edited): "http://en.wikipedia.org/wiki/Occlusion_miliaria"

Occupational acne

Occupational acne is caused by several different groups of industrial compounds, including coal tar derivatives, insoluble cutting oils, and chlorinated hydrocarbons (chlornaphthalenes, chlordiphenyls, and chlordiphenyloxides).
Source (edited): "http://en.wikipedia.org/wiki/Occupational_acne"

Ocular rosacea

Ocular rosacea is a manifestation of rosacea that affects the eyes and eyelids. Symptoms generally consist of redness, irritation or burning of the eyes. Patients may also feel that there is something, such as an eyelash, in the eye. Commonly patients also show redness of the nose and cheeks.

Patients who suffer from ocular rosacea may be treated with warm compresses, artificial tears and washing the area around the eye with warm water, including the eyelids, to help alleviate symptoms. Additionally, oral antibiotics, typically doxycycline, may be prescribed. Some patients feel that dietary restrictions of caffeine, spicy foods, and Alcoholic beverages may reduce or eliminate symptoms.
Source (edited): "http://en.wikipedia.org/wiki/Ocular_rosacea"

Olmsted syndrome

Olmsted syndrome (also known as "Mutilating palmoplantar keratoderma with periorificial keratotic plaques," "Mutilating palmoplantar keratoderma with periorificial plaques" and "Polykeratosis of Touraine") is a keratoderma of the palms and soles, with flexion deformity of the digits, that begins in infancy.

Treatment with retinoids has been described.
Source (edited): "http://en.wikipedia.org/wiki/Olmsted_syndrome"

Oral florid papillomatosis

Oral florid papillomatosis is a condition characterized by a white mass resembling a cauliflower covering the tongue and extending onto other portions of the mucous membranes. This is a type of verrucous carcinoma.
Source (edited): "http://en.wikipedia.org/wiki/Oral_florid_papillomatosis"

Oral melanosis

Oral melanosis is pigmentation of the oral cavity that tends to occur most frequently in black persons.
Source (edited): "http://en.wikipedia.org/wiki/Oral_melanosis"

Orthostatic purpura

Orthostatic purpura (also known as "Stasis purpura") is a skin condition that results from prolonged standing or even sitting with the legs lowered (as in a bus, airplane, or train), which produced edema and a purpuric eruption on the lower extremities.
Source (edited): "http://en.wikipedia.org/wiki/Orthostatic_purpura"

Osseous choristoma of the tongue

Osseous choristoma of the tongue is a condition characterized by a nodule on the dorsum of the tongue containing mature lamellar bone without osteoblastic or osteoclastic activity.
Source (edited): "http://en.wikipedia.org/wiki/Osseous_choristoma_of_the_tongue"

Osteoma cutis

Osteoma cutis is a cutaneous condition characterized by the presence of bone within the skin in the absence of a preexisting or associated lesion.
Source (edited): "http://en.wikipedia.org/wiki/Osteoma_cutis"

Otophyma

Otophyma is a cauliflower-like swelling of one or both ears.
Source (edited): "http://en.wikipedia.org/wiki/Otophyma"

PUVA lentigines

PUVA lentigines are a cutaneous condition caused by PUVA therapy.
Source (edited): "http://en.wikipedia.org/wiki/PUVA_lentigines"

Pagetoid reticulosis

Pagetoid reticulosis (also known as "Acral mycoses fungoides," "Localized epidermotropic reticulosis," "Mycosis fungoides palmaris et plantaris," "Unilesional mycosis fungoides," and "Woringer–Kolopp disease") is a cutaneous condition, an uncommon lymphoproliferative disorder, sometimes considered a form of mycosis fungoides.
Source (edited): "http://en.wikipedia.org/wiki/Pagetoid_reticulosis"

Painful bruising syndrome

Painful bruising syndrome (also known as "Autoerythrocyte sensitization," "Gardner–Diamond syndrome," and "Psychogenic purpura") is an idiopathic trauma-induced condition seen in young to middle-aged women who sometimes manifest personality disorders.. It is characterized by a distinctive localized purpuric reaction occurring primarily on the legs, face and trunk, with recurring painful ecchymoses variably accompanied by syncope, nausea, vomiting, gastrointestinal and intracranial bleeding.

Patients with autoerythrocyte sensitization can suffer frequent painful bruising around joints and muscles. Because of the rarity of the disorder, there are few methods of support in place for patients. Many patients are labelled with the stigma of having a psychological condition without this having a specifically proven link. There have been cases of painful bruising syndrome reported where there are no additional psychological disorders.

It was characterized in 1955.

Source (edited): "http://en.wikipedia. org/wiki/Painful_bruising_syndrome"

Painful fat herniation

Painful fat herniation (also known as "Painful piezogenic pedal papules" and "Piezogenic papules") is a rare cause of painful feet due to fat herniations through the thin fascial layers of the weight-bearing parts of the heel.

Source (edited): "http://en.wikipedia. org/wiki/Painful_fat_herniation"

Palisaded neutrophilic and granulomatous dermatitis

Palisaded neutrophilic and granulomatous dermaitiitis is usually associated with a well-defined connective tissue disease, lupus erythematosus or rheumatoid arthritis most commonly, and often presents with eroded or ulcerated symmetrically distributed umbilicated papules or nodules on the elbows.

Source (edited): "http://en.wikipedia. org/wiki/Palisaded_neutrophilic_and _granulomatous_dermatitis"

Palmar erythema

Palmar erythema is reddening of the palms at the thenar and hypothenar eminences.

Causes

It is associated with various physiological as well as pathological changes, the principal one of which is portal hypertension. It is also seen in patients with liver dysfunction, such as chronic liver disease (chronic hepatitis), and also in pregnant women. Palmar erythema may also be the result of thyrotoxicosis and dermatoses such as eczema or psoriasis, and is related to deep telangiectasias. It may also be a normal finding.

Because circulating levels of estrogen increase in both cirrhosis and pregnancy, estrogen was thought to be the cause for the increased vascularity. More recently, nitric oxide has been implicated in the pathogenesis of palmar erythema.

Palmar erythema occurs in about 30% of patients with rheumatoid arthritis especially those with elevated hemoglobin levels .

Palmar erythema can also be seen in Coxsackievirus A infection (hand, foot and mouth disease), Rocky Mountain Spotted Fever, and secondary Syphilis. . Source (edited): "http://en.wikipedia. org/wiki/Palmar_erythema"

Palmoplantar keratoderma

Palmoplantar keratodermas are a heterogeneous group of disorders characterized by abnormal thickening of the palms and sole

Autosomal recessive and dominant, X-linked, and acquired forms have all been described.

There are also acquired forms of the condition.

Clinical patterns

Clinically, three distinct patterns of palmoplantar keratoderma may be identified: diffuse, focal, and punctate.:

Diffuse

- **Diffuse palmoplantar keratoderma** is a type of palmoplantar keratoderma that is characterized by an even, thick, symmetric hyperkeratosis over the whole of the palm and sole, usually evident at birth or in the first few months of life. Restated, diffuse palmoplantar keratoderma is an autosomal dominant disorder in which hyperkeratosis is confined to the palms and soles. The two major types can have a similar clinical appearance:
- Diffuse epidermolytic palmoplantar keratoderma (also known as "Palmoplantar keratoderma cum degeneratione granulosa Vörner," and "Vörner's epidermolytic palmoplantar keratoderma") is one of the most common patterns of palmoplantar keratoderma, an autosomal dominant condition that presents within the first few months of life, characterized by a well-demarcated, symmetric thickening of palms and soles, often with a "dirty" snakeskin appearance due to underlying epidermolysis
- Diffuse nonepidermolytic palmoplantar keratoderma (also known as "Diffuse orthohyperkeratotic keratoderma," "Hereditary palmoplantar keratoderma," "Keratosis extremitatum progrediens," "Keratosis palmoplantaris diffusa circumscripta," "Tylosis," and "Unna-Thost disease") is inherited as an autosomal dominant condition and is present from infancy, characterized by a well-demarcated, symmetric, often "waxy" keratoderma involving the whole of the palms and soles

Focal

- Focal palmoplantar keratoderma, a type of palmoplantar keratoderma in which large, compact masses of

keratin develop at sites of recurrent friction, principally on the feet, although also on the palms and other sites, a pattern of calluses that may be discoid (nummular) or linear
- Focal palmoplantar keratoderma with oral mucosal hyperkeratosis (also known as "Hereditary painful callosity syndrome," "Keratosis follicularis," and "Keratosis palmoplantaris nummularis") is an autosomal dominant keratoderma that represents a clinical overlap syndrome with pachyonychia congenita type I but without the classic nail involvement

Punctate

- Punctate palmoplantar keratoderma, a form of palmoplantar keratoderma in which many tiny "raindrop" keratoses involve the palmoplantar surface, skin lesions which may involve the whole of the palmoplantar surface, or may be more restricted in their distribution

Ungrouped

- Palmoplantar keratoderma and spastic paraplegia (also known as "Charcot-Marie-Tooth disease with palmoplantar keratoderma and nail dystrophy") is an autosomal dominant or x-linked dominant condition that begins in early childhood with thick focal keratoderma over the soles and, to a lesser extent, the palms
- Palmoplantar keratoderma of Sybert (also known as "Greither palmoplantar keratoderma," "Keratosis extremitatum hereditaria progrediens," and "Keratosis palmoplantaris transgrediens et progrediens") is an extremely rare autosomal dominant keratoderma with symmetric severe involvement of the whole palmoplantar surface in a glove-and-stocking distribution
- Striate palmoplantar keratoderma (also known as "Acral keratoderma," "Brünauer-Fuhs-Siemens type," "Keratosis palmoplantaris varians," and "Wachters palmoplantar keratoderma") is an autosomal dominant keratoderma principally involving the soles with onset in infancy or the first few years of life
- Striate palmoplantar keratoderma, woolly hair, and left ventricular dilated cardiomyopathy has been described in both autosomal dominant and autosomal recessive forms, but only the recessive forms have a clear association with dilated cardiomyopathy

Genetics

Epidermolytic palmoplantar keratoderma has been associated with keratin 9 and keratin 16.

Nonepidermolytic palmoplantar keratoderma has been associated with keratin 1 and keratin 16.

Source (edited): "http://en.wikipedia.org/wiki/Palmoplantar_keratoderma"

Palmoplantar keratoderma and spastic paraplegia

Palmoplantar keratoderma and spastic paraplegia (also known as "Charcot–Marie–Tooth disease with palmoplantar keratoderma and nail dystrophy") is an autosomal dominant or x-linked dominant condition that begins in early childhood with thick focal keratoderma over the soles and, to a lesser extent, the palms.

Source (edited): "http://en.wikipedia.org/wiki/Palmoplantar_keratoderma_and_spastic_paraplegia"

Palmoplantar keratoderma of Sybert

Palmoplantar keratoderma of Sybert (also known as "Greither palmoplantar keratoderma," "Greither syndrome," "Keratosis extremitatum hereditaria progrediens," "Keratosis palmoplantaris transgrediens et progrediens" "Sybert keratoderma," and "Transgrediens and progrediens palmoplantar keratoderma") is an extremely rare autosomal dominant keratoderma (a skin condition involving horn-like growths) with symmetric severe involvement of the whole palmoplantar surface in a glove-and-stocking distribution.

It was characterized by Aloys Greither in 1952.

It was characterized by Virginia Sybert in 1988.

Source (edited): "http://en.wikipedia.org/wiki/Palmoplantar_keratoderma_of_Sybert"

Pancreatic panniculitis

Pancreatic panniculitis (also known as "Enzymatic panniculitis," "Pancreatic fat necrosis," and "Subcutaneous fat necrosis") is a skin condition most commonly associated with pancreatic carcinoma, and more rarely with anatomic pancreatic abnormalities, pseudocysts, or drug-induced pancreatitis.

Source (edited): "http://en.wikipedia.org/wiki/Pancreatic_panniculitis"

Pansclerotic morphea

Pansclerotic morphea is manifested by sclerosis of the dermis, panniculus, fascia, muscle, and at times, the bone, all causing disabling limitation of motion of joints.
Source (edited): "http://en.wikipedia.org/wiki/Pansclerotic_morphea"

Papular mucinosis of infancy

Papular mucinosis of infancy (also known as "Cutaneous mucinosis of infancy") is a skin condition caused by fibroblasts producing abnormally large amounts of mucopolysaccharides, characterized by skin-colored or translucent papules.
Source (edited): "http://en.wikipedia.org/wiki/Papular_mucinosis_of_infancy"

Papular sarcoid

Papular sarcoid is a cutaneous condition characterized by papules, which are the most common morphology of cutaneous sarcoidosis.
Source (edited): "http://en.wikipedia.org/wiki/Papular_sarcoid"

Papular xanthoma

Papular xanthoma is a cutaneous condition that is a rare form of non-X histiocytosis.
Source (edited): "http://en.wikipedia.org/wiki/Papular_xanthoma"

Papuloerythroderma of Ofuji

Papuloerythroderma of Ofuji is a rare disorder most commonly found in Japan, characterized by pruritic papules that spare the skinfolds, producing bands of uninvolved cutis, creating the so-called deck-chair sign. Frequently there is associated blood eosinophilia. Skin biopsies reveal a dense lymphohistiocytic infiltrate, eosinophils in the papillary dermis, and increased Langerhans cells (S-100 positive). Systemic steroids are the treatment of choice and may result in long-term remissions.

It was characterized in 1984.

Use of PUVA in treatment has been described.
Source (edited): "http://en.wikipedia.org/wiki/Papuloerythroderma_of_Ofuji"

Papulopustular rosacea

Papulopustular rosacea (also known as "Inflammatory rosacea") manifests a strikingly red central face accompanied by erythematous papules often surrounded by a pinpoint pustule.
Source (edited): "http://en.wikipedia.org/wiki/Papulopustular_rosacea"

Paraneoplastic pemphigus

Paraneoplastic pemphigus is an autoimmune disorder that is almost invariably linked to an underlying lymphoproliferative disorder.
Source (edited): "http://en.wikipedia.org/wiki/Paraneoplastic_pemphigus"

Parapsoriasis

Parapsoriasis refers to one of a group of skin disorders that are characterized primarily by their resemblance to psoriasis (red, scaly lesions), rather than by their underlying etiology.

Neoplasms can devleop from parapsoriasis. For example, it can develop into cutaneous T-cell lymphoma.

The term "Parapsoriasis" was formed in 1902.

Classification

The parapsoriasis group, described and debated for nearly a century, has spawned a confusing nomenclature. There are some authors who prefer to limit the term "parapsoriasis" to large- and small-plaque variants only. However, the following classification scheme is now generally accepted:

- Large-plaque parapsoriasis
- Small-plaque parapsoriasis
- Pityriasis lichenoides
  - Pityriasis lichenoides chronica
  - Pityriasis lichenoides et varioliformis acuta
- Lymphomatoid papulosis

Source (edited): "http://en.wikipedia.org/wiki/Parapsoriasis"

Paroxysmal hand hematoma

Paroxysmal hand hematoma (also known as "Achenbach syndrome") is a skin condition characterized by spontaneous focal hemorrhage into the palm or the volar surface of a finger, which results in transitory localized pain, followed by rapid swelling and localized blueish discoloration.

Source (edited): "http://en.wikipedia.org/wiki/Paroxysmal_hand_hematoma"

Partial unilateral lentiginosis

Partial unilateral lentiginosis (also known as "Segmental lentiginosis") is a cutaneous condition characterized by lentigines located on only one half of the body.

Source (edited): "http://en.wikipedia.org/wiki/Partial_unilateral_lentiginosis"

Patch-type granuloma annulare

Patch-type granuloma annulare (also known as "Macular granuloma annulare") is a skin condition of unknown cause, more commonly affecting women between 30 and 70 years of age, characterized by flat or slightly palpable erythematous or red-brown skin lesions.

Source (edited): "http://en.wikipedia.org/wiki/Patch-type_granuloma_annulare"

Peat fire cancer

Peat fire cancer is a cutaneous condition that may develop on the shins of women due to hydrocarbon-fueled heat exposure from coal-fired clothing warmers.

Source (edited): "http://en.wikipedia.org/wiki/Peat_fire_cancer"

Pemphigus erythematosus

Pemphigus erythematosus (also known as "Senear–Usher syndrome") is simply a localized form of pemphigus foliaceus.

Source (edited): "http://en.wikipedia.org/wiki/Pemphigus_erythematosus"

Pemphigus foliaceus

Pemphigus foliaceus is an autoimmune blistering disease of the skin and mucous membranes with characteristic lesions that are scaly, crusted erosions, often on an erythematous base. No clinically apparent mucosal involvement is present even with widespread disease.

If there is an autoimmune IgG buildup in the epidermis, then nearly almost all of the antibodies are aimed against Desmoglein 1. The effect of the antibodies and the immunological pathway is most likely either of three mechanisms:

- Steric hindrance of the Desmoglein 1. The antibody caps off the site for intracellular binding to another keratinocyte.
- Activation of a endocytic pathway. The antibody activates a pathway which causes a internationalization of Desmogleïn 1 which in turn causes a loss of adhesion.
- Disruption of function. In this case the antibody blocks the Desmoglein 1 from being formed into a desmosome. This in turn causes a loss of adhesion with acantholysis as a result.

Source (edited): "http://en.wikipedia.org/wiki/Pemphigus_foliaceus"

Pemphigus vegetans

Pemphigus vegetans is a localized form of pemphigus vulgaris. in which there is a localized vegetating papillomatous response. The eroded areas do not heal like usual but form papillomatous growth and vegetation.

Accounts for 1-2% of pemphigus cases and is a relatively benign variant of Pemphigus Vulgaris. Two forms are recognized:

- Neumann type: more common and characterized by early lesions similar to Pemphigus Vulgaris with large bullae and erosive areas. Healing is through formation of granulation tissue.
- Hallopeau type: less aggressive and has pustules not bullae. These pustules heal by verrucios hyperkeratotic vegetations.

Source (edited): "http://en.wikipedia.org/wiki/Pemphigus_vegetans"

Pemphigus vegetans of Hallopeau

Pemphigus vegetans of Hallopeau is a disease of localized pemphigus vulgaris.

It is named for François Henri Hallopeau.

Source (edited): "http://en.wikipedia.org/wiki/Pemphigus_vegetans_of_Hallopeau"

Pemphigus vegetans of Neumann

Pemphigus vegetans of Neumann is a localized disease of pemphigus vulgaris slightly more extensive than pemphigus vegetans of Hallopeau.

Source (edited): "http://en.wikipedia.org/wiki/Pemphigus_vegetans_of_Neumann"

Pemphigus vulgaris

Pemphigus vulgaris is a chronic blistering skin disease with skin lesions that are rarely pruritic, but which are often painful.

Pathophysiology

It is an autoimmune disease caused by antibodies directed against both desmoglein 1 and desmoglein 3 resulting in the loss of cohesion between keratinocytes in the epidermis. It is characterized by extensive flaccid blisters and mucocutaneous erosions. The severity of the disease, as well as the mucosal lesions, is believed to be directly proportional to the levels of desmoglein 3. Milder forms of pemphigus (like foliacious and erythematoses) are more desmoglein 1 heavy. It arises most often in middle-aged or older people, usually starting with a blister that ruptures easily. The lesions can become quite extensive. The pathogenesis of the disease involves autoantibodies against desmosome proteins, separating keratinocytes from the basal layer of the epidermis. On histology, the basal keratinocytes are usually still attached to the basement membrane leading to the appearance and thus the term, "tombstoning".

Transudative fluid accumulates in between the keratinocytes and basement membrane (suprabasal split), forming a blister. This is a contrasting feature from bullous pemphigoid, where the detachment occurs between the epidermis and dermis (subepidermal bullae).

Diagnosis

The gold standard for diagnosis is a punch biopsy of the lesion with direct immunofluorescent staining, showing acantholytic cells. These can also be seen on a Tzanck smear. These cells are basically rounded, nucleated keratinocytes formed due to antibody mediated damage to cell adhesion protein: Desmoglein.

Pemphigus vulgaris is easy to confuse with impetigo and candidiasis. IgG4 is considered pathogenic. The diagnosis can be confirmed by testing for the infections that cause these other conditions, and by a lack of response to antibiotic treatment.

Treatment

Corticosteroids and other immunosuppressive drugs are the mainstay of treatment. Based on recent studies, corticosteroids can be used in Pulse Therapy/ Supra-pharmacological doses once a month to decrease Hypothalamo-pituitary axis inhibition. IVIG, rituximab, cellcept, methotrexate, imuran, and cytoxan have also been used with varying degrees of success. It is a difficult disease to control.

Source (edited): "http://en.wikipedia.org/wiki/Pemphigus_vulgaris"

Perforating calcific elastosis

Perforating calcific elastosis (also known as "Localized acquired cutaneous pseudoxanthoma elasticum," "Perforating periumbilical calcific elastosis," and "Periumbilical perforating pseudoxanthoma elasticum") is an acquired, localized cutaneous disorder, most frequently found in obese, multiparous, middle-aged women, characterized by lax, well-circumscribed, reticulated or cobble-stoned plaques occurring in the periumbilical region with keratotic surface papules.
Source (edited): "http://en.wikipedia.org/wiki/Perforating_calcific_elastosis"

Perforating granuloma annulare

Perforating granuloma annulare is a skin condition of unknown cause, usually appearing on the dorsal hands, presenting as papules with a central keratotic core.
Source (edited): "http://en.wikipedia.org/wiki/Perforating_granuloma_annulare"

Perifolliculitis capitis abscedens et suffodiens

Perifolliculitis capitis abscedens et suffodiens (also known as "Perifolliculitis capitis abscedens et suffodiens of Hoffman," "Dissecting folliculitis," and "Dissecting cellulitis of the scalp") is an inflammatory condition of the scalp that can lead to scarring alopecia, which begins with deep inflammatory nodules, primarily over occiput, that progresses to coalescing regions of boggy scalp.
Source (edited): "http://en.wikipedia.org/wiki/Perifolliculitis_capitis_abscedens_et_suffodiens"

Perinatal gangrene of the buttock

Perinatal gangrene of the buttock is a skin condition similar to livedoid dermatitis, and is usually a complication of umbilical artery catheterization, exchange transfusion, or cord injections by means of a syringe.
Source (edited): "http://en.wikipedia.org/wiki/Perinatal_gangrene_of_the_buttock"

Perioral dermatitis

Perioral dermatitis, a condition related to acne vulgaris, consists of red papules that may appear microvesicular that typically affect the nasolabial folds (around the nostrils), perioral area (around the mouth) or perioccular area (around the eyes). It usually affects women between the ages of 20 and 45. It is not uncommon, and has a tendency to recur in individuals who have had it once.

Causes

It is commonly caused by the use of fluorinated topical glucocorticoid steroids to this area, although it can have many other causes, including fluoride toothpastes or simply continual irritation. It is exacerbated by cosmetics, soaps, facial washes and steroid creams so use of these things on the affected area is not advisable.

Treatment

It is treated in a similar manner to acne vulgaris with tetracycline antibiotics or erythromycin but without the use of topical steroids.
Source (edited): "http://en.wikipedia.org/wiki/Perioral_dermatitis"

Periorbital dermatitis

Periorbital dermatitis (also known as "Periocular dermatitis") is a skin condition, a variant of perioral dermatitis, occurring on the lower eyelids and skin adjacent to the upper and lower eyelids.
Source (edited): "http://en.wikipedia.org/wiki/Periorbital_dermatitis"

Periorbital hyperpigmentation

Periorbital hyperpigmentation is characterized by dark circles around the eyes, which are common, often familial, and frequently found in individuals with dark pigmentation or Mediterranean ancestry. Atopic patients may also exhibit periorbital pigmentation (allergic shiners), and treatment is ineffective.

Source (edited): "http://en.wikipedia.org/wiki/Periorbital_hyperpigmentation"

Persistent edema of rosacea

Persistent edema of rosacea (also known as "Chronic upper facial erythematous edema," "Morbihan's disease," or "Rosaceous lymphedema") is a hard, nonpitting edema found on the areas involved, those mainly being the forehard, glabella, upper eyelids, nose, and/or cheeks.

Persistent edema of rosacea is an uncommon cutaneous condition characterized by a hard, nonpitting edema restricted to the forehead, glabella, upper eyelids, nose, and cheeks. This condition is also known as chronic upper facial erythematous edema, Morbihan's disease, morbus Morbihan, and rosaceous lymphedema. Despite the name, it is unclear whether this condition is a distinct disease or a rare complication of rosacea. Generally, there are few symptomatic complaints aside from redness and facial contour changes. The edema typically worsens slowly over months to years and is often on a background of chronic inflammation. There are no specific laboratory findings associated with this condition, and the histology tends to be similar to that seen in rosacea. The differential diagnosis includes acne vulgaris, streptococcal cellulitis, and Melkersson–Rosenthal syndrome, as these conditions can also rarely manifest with a similar edema, as well as other forms of rosacea, lupus erythematosus, and sarcoidosis.

Most cases of this condition tend to be recalcitrant to treatment, with topical and oral antibiotic regiments commonly used for rosacea generally being ineffective. For the severe forms of this disease, oral isotretinoin therapy has been used, and the condition responds well to doses of 0.5 to 1 mg/kg/day. However, unlike in the treatment of acne vulgaris, lasting responses to isotretinoin generally do not occur, and long-term maintenance therapy with oral tetracyclines is usually necessary. Eyelid reduction surgery has also been reported to help with the cosmetic appearance of the condition, but does not alter the disease progression.

Source (edited): "http://en.wikipedia.org/wiki/Persistent_edema_of_rosacea"

Photoaging

Photoaging (also known as "Dermatoheliosis") is a term used for the characteristic changes induced by chronic UVA and UVB exposure. Tretinoin is the best studied retinoid in the treatment of photoaging

Source (edited): "http://en.wikipedia.org/wiki/Photoaging"

Photodermatosis

Photodermatosis is a skin disease that is caused by exposure to sunlight.

People with photodermatosis may develop skin rashes following exposure to the sun. Polymorphous Light Eruption is the most common type of photodermatosis. It is most likely due to an abnormal immune system reaction to the sun. Polymorphous light eruption occurs in approximately 10 to 20 percent of otherwise healthy individuals, so it is a relatively common condition.

Source (edited): "http://en.wikipedia.org/wiki/Photodermatosis"

Photosensitive drug reaction

Photosensitive drug reaction (or **drug-induced photosensitivity**) secondary to medications may cause phototoxic, photoallergic, and lichenoid reactions, and photodistributed telangiectasias, as well as pseudoporphyria.

Drugs involved include naproxen and doxycycline.

Source (edited): "http://en.wikipedia.org/wiki/Photosensitive_drug_reaction"

Photosensitivity with HIV infection

Photosensitivity with HIV infection is a skin condition resembling polymorphous light eruption, actinic prurigo, or chronic actinic dermatitis, seen in about 5% of HIV-infected people.

Source (edited): "http://en.wikipedia.org/wiki/Photosensitivity_with_HIV_infection"

Phototoxic tar dermatitis

Phototoxic tar dermatitis results from coal tar, creosote, crude coal tar, or pitch, in conjunction with sunlight exposure, which induces a sunburn reaction associated with severe burning sensation.

Source (edited): "http://en.wikipedia.org/wiki/Phototoxic_tar_dermatitis"

Phymatous rosacea

Phymatous rosacea is a cutaneous condition characterized by overgrowth of sebaceous glands. "Phyma" is the Greek word for swelling, mass, or bulb, and these can occur in various areas of the face and ears in associated with rosacea. Types of phyma seen in rosacea are:

- Rhinophyma
- Gnathophyma
- Metophyma
- Otophyma
- Blepharophyma

Source (edited): "http://en.wikipedia.org/wiki/Phymatous_rosacea"

Pigmentation disorder

Pigmentation disorders are disturbances of human skin color, either loss or reduction, which may be related to loss of melanocytes or the inability of melanocytes to produce melanin or transport melanosomes correctly.

Source (edited): "http://en.wikipedia.org/wiki/Pigmentation_disorder"

Pigmented purpuric dermatosis

Pigmented purpuric dermatosis (also known as "progressive pigmentary dermatosis," "purpura pigmentosa chronica," "pigmentary purpuric eruptions," or "progressive pigmenting purpura") refers to one of the three major classes of skin conditions characterized by purpuric skin eruptions.

Pigmented purpuric dermatosis are distinguished from other purpura by size (0.3-1 cm) and are most often seen in the lower extremities. Pigmentary purpuric eruptions may present with one of several clinical patterns. There may be overlapping characteristics among pigmented purpuric dermatosis and between their signs and those of other purpuric eruptions. Examples of the pigmented purpuric dermatosis group include:

- Schamberg's disease
- Majocchi's disease (Purpura annularis telangiectodes)
- Gougerot-Blum syndrome (Pigmented purpuric lichenoid dermatitis)
- Ducas and Kapetanakis pigmented purpura
- Lichen aureus

Although vascular damage may be present, it is insufficient for these conditions to be considered forms of vasculitis.

Source (edited): "http://en.wikipedia.org/wiki/Pigmented_purpuric_dermatosis"

Plasma cell cheilitis

Plasma cell cheilitis (also known as "Plasma cell gingivitis," and "Plasma cell orificial mucositi") is a condition characterized by a sharply outlined, infiltrated, dark red plaque with a lacquer-like glazing of the surface of the involved oral area.

Source (edited): "http://en.wikipedia.org/wiki/Plasma_cell_cheilitis"

Plasmoacanthoma

Plasmoacanthoma is a condition of the oral mucosa characterized by a verrucous tumor with a plasma cell infiltrate.

Source (edited): "http://en.wikipedia.org/wiki/Plasmoacanthoma"

Pleomorphic T-cell lymphoma

Pleomorphic T-cell lymphoma (also known as "Non-mycosis fungoides CD30− pleomorphic small/medium sized cutaneous T-cell lymphoma") is a cutaneous condition characterized by a 5-year survival rate of 62%.

Source (edited): "http://en.wikipedia.org/wiki/Pleomorphic_T-cell_lymphoma"

Polypoid melanoma

Polypoid melanoma is a rare cutaneous condition, a virulent variant of nodular melanoma.
Source (edited): "http://en.wikipedia.org/wiki/Polypoid_melanoma"

Pomade acne

Pomade acne occurs when some of the pomade that is applied to the scalp is also applied to the forehead and is responsible for the development of multiple, closely packed comedones close to the hairline.

Source (edited): "http://en.wikipedia.org/wiki/Pomade_acne"

Porokeratosis plantaris discreta

Porokeratosis plantaris discreta is a skin condition that occurs in adults, with a 4:1 female preponderance, characterized by a sharply marginated, rubbery, wide-based papule.

It is also known as "Steinberg's lesion".

It was characterized in 1970.

Source (edited): "http://en.wikipedia.org/wiki/Porokeratosis_plantaris_discreta"

Porokeratosis punctata palmaris et plantaris

Spiny keratoderma (also known as "Porokeratosis punctata palmaris et plantaris," "Punctate keratoderma," and "Punctate porokeratosis of the palms and soles") is an autosomal dominant keratoderma of late onset that develops in patients aged 12 to 50, characterized by multiple tiny keratotic plugs, mimicking the spines on a music box, involving the entire palmoplantar surfaces.

Source (edited): "http://en.wikipedia.org/wiki/Porokeratosis_punctata_palmaris_et_plantaris"

Post-steroid panniculitis

Post-steroid panniculitis is a skin condition characterized by inflammation of the subcutaneous fat occurring predominantly in children treated acutely with high doses of systemic corticosteroids during rapid corticosteroid withdrawal.

Source (edited): "http://en.wikipedia.org/wiki/Post-steroid_panniculitis"

Postcardiotomy syndrome

Postcardiotomy syndrome occurs two to three weeks (up to one year) after pericardiotomy, and is characterized by fever, pleuritis, pericarditis, or arthritis, together with petechiae on the skin and palate.. The cause is believed to be an autoimmune response against damaged cardiac tissue. This is supported by excellent response to immunosuppressive (steroid) therapy.

Source (edited): "http://en.wikipedia.org/wiki/Postcardiotomy_syndrome"

Postencephalitic trophic ulcer

Postencephalitic trophic ulcer is an ulceration of the nose similar to trigeminal trophic lesions, and has been reported following epidemic encephalitis and herpes zoster of the trigeminal nerve.
Source (edited): "http://en.wikipedia.org/wiki/Postencephalitic_trophic_ulcer"

Postinflammatory hyperpigmentation

Postinflammatory hyperpigmentation (also known as "Postinflammatory hypermelanosis") can result from any natural or iatrogenic inflammatory condition, resulting from two mechanism: (1) increased epidermal pigmentation

via increased melanocyte activity or (2) dermal melanosis from melanocyte damage and melanin drop out from the epidermis into the dermis.
Source (edited): "http://en.wikipedia.org/wiki/Postinflammatory_hyperpigmentation"

Postinflammatory hypopigmentation

Postinflammatory hypopigmentation is a cutaneous condition characterized by decreased pigment in the skin following inflammation of the skin.
Source (edited): "http://en.wikipedia.org/wiki/Postinflammatory_hypopigmentation"

Postinflammatory lymphedema

Postinflammatory lymphedema is a condition characterized by swelling of the soft tissues in which an excessive amount of lymph has accumulated, and is caused by repeated bacterial infections.
Source (edited): "http://en.wikipedia.org/wiki/Postinflammatory_lymphedema"

Postmiliarial hypohidrosis

Postmiliarial hypohidrosis is a skin condition that results from occlusion of sweat ducts and pores, and may be severe enough to impair an individual's ability to perform sustained work in a hot environment.
Source (edited): "http://en.wikipedia.org/wiki/Postmiliarial_hypohidrosis"

Pressure urticaria

Pressure urticaria (also known as **delayed pressure urticaria**) is a physical urticaria caused by pressure applied to the skin, and is characterized by the development of swelling and pain that usually occurs 3 to 12 hours after local pressure has been applied.
Source (edited): "http://en.wikipedia.org/wiki/Pressure_urticaria"

Primary cutaneous follicular lymphoma

Primary cutaneous follicular lymphoma (also known as "Follicular center cell lymphoma," and "Follicular center lymphoma") is a cutaneous condition characterized by single or multiple papules, plaques or nodules with surrounding erythema.
Source (edited): "http://en.wikipedia.org/wiki/Primary_cutaneous_follicular_lymphoma"

Primary cutaneous immunocytoma

Primary cutaneous immunocytoma is a skin condition that represents a low grade B-cell lymphoma related to marginal zone B-cell lymphoma but with a predominance of cells having plasmacytic features.
Source (edited): "http://en.wikipedia.org/wiki/Primary_cutaneous_immunocytoma"

Primary cutaneous marginal zone lymphoma

Primary cutaneous marginal zone lymphomas represent a heterogeneous group of diseases characterized by solitary or multiple dermal or subcutaneous nodules. Lymphomas included in this group are:

- Primary cutaneous immunocytoma
- Marginal zone B-cell lymphoma
- Mucosa-associated lymphoid tissue lymphoma

Source (edited): "http://en.wikipedia.org/wiki/Primary_cutaneous_marginal_zone_lymphoma"

Primary systemic amyloidosis

Primary systemic amyloidosis is a disease that involves the mesenchymal tissue, the tongue, heart, gastrointestinal tract, and skin.
Source (edited): "http://en.wikipedia.org/wiki/Primary_systemic_amyloidosis"

Prion pruritus

Prion pruritus is the intense itching during the prodromal period of the Creutzfeldt-Jakob disease.
Source (edited): "http://en.wikipedia.org/wiki/Prion_pruritus"

Progressive nodular histiocytosis

Progressive nodular histiocytosis is a cutaneous condition clinically characterized by the development of two types of skin lesions: superficial papules and deeper larger subcutaneous nodules.
Source (edited): "http://en.wikipedia.org/wiki/Progressive_nodular_histiocytosis"

Progressive systemic sclerosis

Progressive systemic sclerosis is a generalized disorder of connective tissue in which there is thickening of dermal collagen bundles, and fibrosis and vascular abnormalities in internal organs.
Source (edited): "http://en.wikipedia.org/wiki/Progressive_systemic_sclerosis"

Proliferative verrucous leukoplakia

Proliferative verrucous leukoplakia is a slowly progressive condition characterized by thickened and enlarged sites of oral mucous membrane.
Source (edited): "http://en.wikipedia.org/wiki/Proliferative_verrucous_leukoplakia"

Prurigo gestationis

Prurigo gestationis (also called "Besnier prurigo", "Early-onset prurigo of pregnancy," "Linear IgM dermatosis of pregnancy," "Papular dermatitis of pregnancy," "Prurigo of pregnancy", and "Spangler's papular dermatitis of pregnancy") is an eruption consisting of pruritic, excoriated papules of the proximal limbs and upper trunk, most often occurring between the 20th and 34th week of gestation.

The exact etiology is unknown, but it is considered likely to be a flareup of atopic dermatitis during pregnancy.

It is sometimes considered to be a term encompassing Besnier prurigo and other conditions.

It is sometimes considered a diagnosis of exclusion.
Source (edited): "http://en.wikipedia.org/wiki/Prurigo_gestationis"

Prurigo pigmentosa

Prurigo pigmentosa is a rare skin condition of unknown cause, characterized by the sudden onset of erythematous papules that leave a reticulated hyperpigmentation when they heal.
Source (edited): "http://en.wikipedia.org/wiki/Prurigo_pigmentosa"

Prurigo simplex

Prurigo simplex is a term for a chronic, itchy, idiopathic skin condition.
Source (edited): "http://en.wikipedia.org/wiki/Prurigo_simplex"

Pruritic folliculitis of pregnancy

Pruritic folliculitis of pregnancy is a dermatosis of pregnancy characterized by small follicular pustules scattered widely over the trunk, appearing during the second or third trimester, and resolving by 2 or 3 weeks after delivery.

Source (edited): "http://en.wikipedia.org/wiki/Pruritic_folliculitis_of_pregnancy"

Pruritus scroti

Pruritus scroti is itchiness of the scrotum that may be secondary to an infectious cause.

Source (edited): "http://en.wikipedia.org/wiki/Pruritus_scroti"

Pruritus vulvae

Pruritus vulvae is pruritus of the vulva, which is the counterpart of pruritus scroti, and may be caused by many different causes.

Causes

This condition is a symptom of an underlying condition more often than it is a primary condition. Vulva irritation can be caused by any moisture left on the skin. This moisture may be perspiration, urine, vaginal discharge or small amounts of stool. It may be caused by vaginal infections, vulvitis, HPV (Human Papilloma Virus) infection, anal incontinence, Bowen's disease, or dietary irritants (caffeine, tomatoes, and peanuts).

Treatment with antibiotics can lead to a yeast infection and irritation of the vulva. Some diseases increase the possibility of yeast infections, such as diabetes mellitus or HIV infection.

Chronic inflammation of the vulva predisposes to the development of premalignant or malignant changes.

Source (edited): "http://en.wikipedia.org/wiki/Pruritus_vulvae"

Pseudoporphyria

Pseudoporphyria (also known as "Pseudoporphyria cutanea tarda") is a bullous photosensitivity that clinically and histologically mimics porphyria cutanea tarda. The difference is that no abnormalities in urine or serum porphyrin is noted on laboratories. Pseudoporphyria has been reported in patients with chronic renal failure treated with hemodialysis and in those with excessive exposure to ultraviolet A (UV-A) by tanning beds.

Pathophysiology

The precise pathophysiologic mechanism of pseudoporphyria is not fully understood. Some drugs, especially non steroidal anti-inflammatory drugs, can trigger pseudoporphyria in the presence of ultraviolet light.

The pathophysiology of pseudoporphyria associated with hemodialysis has not been fully explained. Aluminum hydroxide has been implicated in hemodialysis-associated pseudoporphyria. Aluminum hydroxide is found in dialysis solution and has been shown to produce a porphyrialike disorder after long-term administration in rats.

Frequency

Although fewer than 100 cases are documented in English language literature, pseudoporphyria is most likely underreported in the literature because it is only a symptom of some other affliction, e.g. side effect of medicine or symptom of liver problems. As the symptoms of pseudoporhphyra have other names, those symptoms are mentioned .

The rarity of porphyria in modern times also makes the use of the term pseudoporphyria obscure.

Race

Although pseudoporphyria has no predilection toward any one race, it has been shown that fair-skinned children who are highly prone to sunburn are more likely to develop naproxen-induced pseudoporphyria than those children with skin types III or higher. Wallace et al. demonstrated that even in the absence of a history of blistering, children with light skin and blue or green eyes are at an increased risk of developing shallow scars on the face while taking naproxen.

History

A careful history is of utmost importance when the diagnosis of pseudoporphyria is being considered. A personal and family history of hepatitis, porphyria, or photosensitivity disorder must be sought. Although a genetic factor has not been considered in pseudoporphyria, one case of monozygotic twins developing pseudoporphyria after excessive UV-A exposure from long-term tanning bed use has been documented. The patient should be thoroughly questioned regarding any symptoms of connective tissue disorder, which may be the underlying pathology of the photosensitivity. Recent reports suggest that a connective tissue disorder may be a predisposing factor in patients using nonsteroidal anti-inflammatory drugs (NSAIDs) who develop pseudoporphyria.

Physical Findings

Pseudoporphyria is clinically characterized by increased skin fragility; erythema; and the appearance of tense bullae and erosions on sun-exposed skin, which are identical to those seen in patients with PCT. However, a clinical pearl that may prove helpful in differentiating between pseudoporphyria and PCT is that the classic features of hypertrichosis, hyperpigmentation, and sclerodermoid changes found with PCT are unusual with pseudoporphyria. A second clinical pattern of pseudoporphyria has a similar presentation to erythropoietic protoporphyria (EPP), an autosomal dominant porphyria resulting from a reduced activity of ferrochelatase.

In contrast to PCT, EPP usually begins in childhood with a history of photosensitivity, often described as a burning sensation immediately after sunlight exposure. Clinically, EPP is characterized by erythema, edema, shallow scars, and waxy induration of the skin, particularly on the face. Pseudoporphyria that clinically mimics EPP has been described almost exclusively in children taking naproxen for juvenile rheumatoid arthritis. Naproxen-induced pseudoporphyria seems to have a dimorphic presentation with the PCT-like pattern more often seen in the adult population and the EPP-like pattern more commonly seen in children, although some overlap has been documented.

Causes

Pseudoporphyria can be induced by a wide range of medications, excessive UV-A exposure, and hemodialysis. One frequently reported drug is naproxen. A frequent source of UV-A exposure is tanning booths.

As recognition of pseudoporphyria increases and the number of new medications expands, the list of etiologic agents associated with pseudoporphyria will most likely continue to grow. Agents associated with pseudoporphyria are as follows :

Propionic acid derivatives (NSAIDs) - naproxen, diflunisal, ketoprofen, nabumetone, oxaprozin, mefenamic acid, rofecoxib

Antibiotics - nalidixic acid, tetracycline, oxytetracycline, ampicillin-sulbactam, cefepime, fluoroquinolones (M Poh, personal communication, June 1999)

Antifungals - voriconazole

Diuretics - furosemide, chlorthalidone, butamide, triamterene/hydrochlorothiazide

Antiarrhythmics - amiodarone

Chemotherapy - 5-fluorouracil

Immunosuppressants - cyclosporine

Sulfones - dapsone

Vitamins - brewers' yeast, pyridoxine

Vitamin A derivatives - etretinate, isotretinoin

Muscle relaxants - carisoprodol/aspirin

Nonsteroidal antiandrogens - flutamide

Other - hemodialysis, excessive UV-A, cola, oral contraceptive pills (levonorgestrel and ethinyl estradiol), narrowband UV-B phototherapy (rarely)

Treatment

Sun avoidance, avoidance of tanning booths, and usage of broad spectrum sunscreen that blocks both UVA and UVB.

Identification and avoidance of the offending drug.

Source (edited): "http://en.wikipedia.org/wiki/Pseudoporphyria"

Pseudoverrucous papules and nodules

Pseudoverrucous papules and nodules are a skin condition characterized by striking 2- to 8-mm, shiny, smooth, red, moist, flat-topped, round skin lesions in the perianal area of children.

Source (edited): "http://en.wikipedia.org/wiki/Pseudoverrucous_papules_and_nodules"

Psoriatic erythroderma

Psoriatic erythroderma (also known as "Erythrodermic psoriasis") represents a generalized form of psoriasis that affects all body sites, including the face, hands, feet, nails, trunk, and extremities.

Source (edited): "http://en.wikipedia.org/wiki/Psoriatic_erythroderma"

Psychogenic pruritus

Psychogenic pruritus is a common manifestation of chronic anxiety, usually a localized itch, especially in the anogenital area.

Source (edited): "http://en.wikipedia.org/wiki/Psychogenic_pruritus"

Puncta pruritica

Puncta pruritica (also known as "Itchy points") consists of one or two itchy spots in clinically normal skin, sometimes followed by the appearance of seborrheic keratoses at exactly the same site.

Source (edited): "http://en.wikipedia. org/wiki/Puncta_pruritica"

Punctate palmoplantar keratoderma

Punctate palmoplantar keratoderma (or **palmoplantar punctate keratoderma**) is a form of palmoplantar keratoderma in which many tiny "raindrop" keratoses involve the palmoplantar surface, skin lesions which may involve the whole of the palmoplantar surface, or may be more restricted in their distribution.

- Type 1: Keratosis punctata palmaris et plantaris
- Type 2: Porokeratosis punctata palmaris et plantaris
- Type 3: Acrokeratoelastoidosis

Source (edited): "http://en.wikipedia. org/wiki/Punctate_palmoplantar_keratoderma"

Purpura fulminans

Purpura fulminans (also known as "Purpura gangrenosa") is a haemorrhagic condition usually associated with sepsis or previous infection. It occurs mainly in babies and small children.

It was first described by Guelliot in 1884.

Presentation

It is a life-threatening disorder of acute onset. It is characterized by cutaneous haemorrhage and necrosis (tissue death), low blood pressure, fever and disseminated intravascular coagulation.

Causes

Common causes are severe infection (especially with meningococcus, and *Capnocytophaga canimorsus*, and other Gram-negative organisms), and deficiency of the natural anticoagulants protein C or protein S in the blood. In some cases, a cause is never found.

Treatment

Treatment is mainly by removing the underlying cause and degree of clotting abnormalities and with supportive treatment (antibiotics, volumne expansion, tissue oxygenation, etc). Thus, treatment includes agressive management of the septic state. Surgical debridement, escharotomies, fasciotomies, and even amputations. In many cases, digits may need to be amputated when their blood supply has ceased completely. Drotrecogin alfa has been recommended for use as ajuvant therapy in some patients. The use of full dose heparin or other anticoagulant is controversial.

Source (edited): "http://en.wikipedia. org/wiki/Purpura_fulminans"

Purpura secondary to clotting disorders

Purpura secondary to clotting disorders are purpura (red or purple discolorations on the skin) which occur due to hereditary disorders of blood coagulation in which there is a deficiency or qualitative abnormality of a single coagulation factor, as in hemophilia or von Willebrand's disease.

Source (edited): "http://en.wikipedia. org/wiki/Purpura_secondary_to_clotting_disorders"

Purpuric agave dermatitis

Purpuric agave dermatitis is a skin condition condition caused by *Agave americana*, a large, thick, long-leaved, subtropical plant.

Source (edited): "http://en.wikipedia. org/wiki/Purpuric_agave_dermatitis"

Pustular bacterid

Pustular bacterid is a skin condition characterized by a symmetric, grouped, vesicular or pustular eruption on the palms and soles marked by exacerbations and remissions over long periods of time.

Source (edited): "http://en.wikipedia. org/wiki/Pustular_bacterid"

Pustulosis

Pustulosis is highly inflammatory skin condition resulting in large fluid-filled blister-like areas - pustules. Pustulosis typically occurs on the palms of the hands and/or the soles of the feet. The skin of these areas peels and flakes (exfoliates). This condition- also referred to as "palmo-plantar pustulosis" - is a feature of pustular psoriasis.

Source (edited): "http://en.wikipedia. org/wiki/Pustulosis"

Pustulosis palmaris et plantaris

Pustulosis palmaris et plantaris (also known as "Pustulosis of palms and soles," "Palmoplantar pustulosis," "Persistent palmoplantar pustulosis," "Pustular psoriasis of the Barber type," and "Pustular psoriasis of the extremities") is a chronic recurrent pustular dermatosis localized on the palms and soles only, characterized histologically by intraepidermal vesicles filled with neutrophils.

Source (edited): "http://en.wikipedia. org/wiki/Pustulosis_palmaris_et_plantaris"

Pyoderma faciale

Pyoderma faciale (also known as "Rosacea fulminans") is a conglobate, nodular disease springing up abruptly on the face.

Source (edited): "http://en.wikipedia. org/wiki/Pyoderma_faciale"

Pyoderma gangrenosum

Pyoderma gangrenosum is a disease that causes tissue to become necrotic, causing deep ulcers that usually occur on the legs. When they occur, they can lead to chronic wounds. Ulcers usually initially look like small bug bites or papules, and they progress to larger ulcers. Though the wounds rarely lead to death, they can cause pain and scarring.

The disease was identified in 1930. It affects approximately 1 person in 100,000 in the population. Though it can affect people of any age, it mostly affects people in their 40s and 50s.

Types

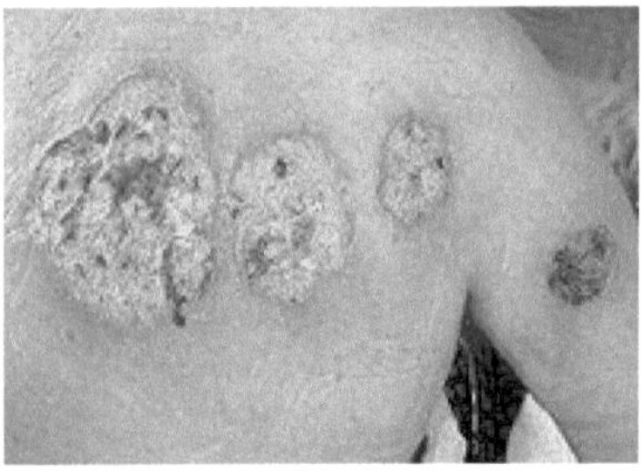

Pyoderma gangrenosum

There are two main types of pyoderma gangrenosum:

- the 'typical' ulcerative form, which occurs in the legs
- an 'atypical' form that is more superficial and occurs in the hands and other parts of the body

Other variations are:

- Peristomal pyoderma gangrenosum is 15% of all cases of pyoderma
- Bullous pyoderma gangrenosum
- Pustular pyoderma gangrenosum
- Vegetative pyoderma gangrenosum

Causes

Though the etiology is not well understood, the disease is thought to be due to immune system dysfunction, and particularly improper functioning of neutrophils. At least half of all pyoderma gangrenosum patients also suffer from illnesses that affect their systemic function. For instance, ulcerative colitis, Crohn's disease, rheumatoid arthritis, and multiple myeloma (MM) sufferers have the condition. It can also be part of a syndrome, for instance in PAPA syndrome. Major and minor trauma are also believed to play a role.

Associations

The common conditions associated with pyoderma gangrenosum are:

- Inflammatory bowel disease:
  - Ulcerative colitis
  - Crohn's disease
- Arthritides:
  - Rheumatoid arthritis
  - Seronegative symmetrical polyarthritis
- Haematological disease:
  - Myelocytic leukemia
  - Hairy cell leukemia
  - Myelofibrosis
  - Myeloid metaplasia
  - Monoclonal gammopathy (IgA)

Treatment

First-line therapy for disseminated or localized instances of pyoderma gangrenosum is systemic treatment by corticosteroids and cyclosporine. If ineffective, alternative therapeutic procedures include systemic treatment with corticosteroids and mycophenolate mofetil; mycophenolate mofetil and cyclosporine; tacrolimus; thalidomide; infliximab; or plasmapheresis.

Source (edited): "http://en.wikipedia. org/wiki/Pyoderma_gangrenosum"

Pyostomatitis vegetans

Pyostomatitis vegetans is an inflammatory stomatitis and most often seen in association with ulcerative colitis.

Source (edited): "http://en.wikipedia. org/wiki/Pyostomatitis_vegetans"

Quadrichrome vitiligo

Quadrichrome vitiligo is another variant of vitiligo, a cutaneous condition, which reflects the presence of a fourth color (dark brown) at sites of perifollicular repigmentation.

Source (edited): "http://en.wikipedia.org/wiki/Quadrichrome_vitiligo"

Radiation acne

Radiation acne is a cutaneous condition characterized by comedo-like papules occurring at sites of previous exposure to therapeutic ionizing radiation, skin lesions that begin to appear as the acute phase of radiation dermatitis begins to resolve.

Source (edited): "http://en.wikipedia.org/wiki/Radiation_acne"

Radiation cancer

Radiation cancer may occur following ionizing radiation exposure following a latent period averaging 20 to 40 years. Various malignancies may develop, most frequency basal-cell carcinoma followed by squamous-cell carcinoma. Elevated risk is confined to the site of radiation exposure. Several studies have also suggested the possibility of a causal relationship between melanoma and ionizing radiation exposure. The degree of carcinogenic risk arising from low levels of exposure is more contentious, but the available evidence points to an increased risk that is approximately proportional to the dose received. Radiologists and radiologic technologists are among the earliest occupational groups exposed to radiation. It was the observation of the earliest radiologists that led to the recognition of radiation-induced skin cancer—the first solid cancer linked to radiation—in 1902. While the incidence of skin cancer secondary to medical ionizing radiation was higher in the past, there is also some evidence that risks of certain cancers, notably skin cancer, may be increased among more recent medical radiation workers, and this may be related to specific or changing radiologic practices. Available evidence indicates that the excess risk of skin cancer lasts for 45 years or more following irradiation.

Source (edited): "http://en.wikipedia.org/wiki/Radiation_cancer"

Radiation dermatitis

Radiation dermatitis (also known as **radiodermatitis**) is a skin disease associated with prolonged exposure to radiation. Radiation dermatitis occurs to some degree in most patients receiving radiotherapy, with or without chemotherapy.

There are three specific types of radiodermatitis: acute radiodermatitis, chronic radiodermatitis, and eosinophilic, polymorphic, and pruritic eruption associated with radiotherapy. However, radiation therapy may also lead to radiation cancer.

With interventional fluoroscopy, because of the high skin doses that can be generated in the course of the intervention, some procedures have resulted in early (less than two months after exposure) and/or late (two months or more after exposure) skin reactions, including necrosis in some cases.

Radiation dermatitis, in the form of intense erythema and vesiculation of the skin, may be observed in radiation ports.

As many as 95% of patients treated with radiation therapy for cancer will experience a skin reaction. Some reactions are immediate, while others may be later (e.g., months after treatment).

Source (edited): "http://en.wikipedia.org/wiki/Radiation_dermatitis"

Reactive neutrophilic dermatoses

Reactive neutrophilic dermatoses are a spectrum of conditions mediated by neutrophils, and typically associated with underlying diseases, such as inflammatory bowel disease and hematologic malignancy.

Conditions considered to be reactive neutrophilic dermatoses include:

- Erythema nodosum
- Marshall syndrome
- Sweet syndrome (Acute febrile neutrophilic dermatosis)
- Neutrophilic dermatosis of the dorsal hands (Pustular vasculitis of the dorsal hands)
- Neutrophilic eccrine hidradenitis
- Pyoderma gangrenosum
- PAPA syndrome

Source (edited): "http://en.wikipedia.org/wiki/Reactive_neutrophilic_dermatoses"

Reticular erythematous mucinosis

Reticular erythematous mucinosis (REM) — also known as **Midline mucinosis**, **Plaque-like cutaneous mucinosis**, and **REM syndrome** — is a skin condition caused by fibroblasts producing abnormally large amounts of mucopolysaccharides. It is a disease that tends to affect women in the third and fourth decades of life.

Source (edited): "http://en.wikipedia.org/wiki/Reticular_erythematous_mucinosis"

Reticular pigmented anomaly of the flexures

Reticular pigmented anomaly of the flexures (also known as "Dark dot disease," and "Dowling–Degos' disease") is a reticular pigmented anomaly of the flexures, an autosomal-dominant pigmentary disorder appearing in adolescence or adulthood, affecting the axillae, neck, and inframammary/sternal areas. This condition is due to mutations in structural/desmosomal proteins found within stratified squamous epithelium.

It is associated with *KRT5*.

Source (edited): "http://en.wikipedia.org/wiki/Reticular_pigmented_anomaly_of_the_flexures"

Reticulate acropigmentation of Kitamura

Reticulate acropigmentation of Kitamura consists of linear palmar pits and pigmented macules 1 to 4mm in diameter on the volar and dorsal aspects of the hands and feet, usually inherited in an autosomal-dominant fashion.

Source (edited): "http://en.wikipedia.org/wiki/Reticulate_acropigmentation_of_Kitamura"

Reticulohistiocytoma

Reticulohistiocytoma is a cutaneous condition characterized by a solitary, firm, dermal skin lesion of less than 1cm in diameter. It usually occurs in young adults or middle aged people, most commonly in females. Affected regions include the head and neck region and the upper part of the trunk. It may coexist with certain neoplasms or vasculitis, and in 30 percent of patients with xanthelasma.

Source (edited): "http://en.wikipedia.org/wiki/Reticulohistiocytoma"

Reticulohistiocytosis

Reticulohistiocytosis is a cutaneous condition of which there are two distinct forms:

- Reticulohistiocytoma
- Multicentric reticulohistiocytosis

Source (edited): "http://en.wikipedia.org/wiki/Reticulohistiocytosis"

Rheumatoid vasculitis

Rheumatoid vasculitis is skin condition that is a typical feature of rheumatoid arthritis, presenting as peripheral vascular lesions that are localized purpura, cutaneous ulceration, and gangrene of the distal parts of the extremities.

Source (edited): "http://en.wikipedia.org/wiki/Rheumatoid_vasculitis"

Riehl melanosis

Riehl melanosis is a form of contact dermatitis, beginning with pruritus, erythema, and pigmentation that gradually spreads which, after reaching a certain extent, becomes stationary. The pathogenesis of Riehl melanosis is believed to be sun exposire following the use of some perfumes or creams (a photocontact dermatitis).

Source (edited): "http://en.wikipedia.org/wiki/Riehl_melanosis"

Rosacea conglobata

Rosacea conglobata is a severe rosacea that shows a reaction which mimics acne conglobata with hemorrhagic nodular abscesses and indurated plaques.

Source (edited): "http://en.wikipedia.org/wiki/Rosacea_conglobata"

SAHA syndrome

SAHA syndrome is characterized by seborrhoea, acne, hirsutism and alopecia, and was first described in 1982, frequently associated with polycystic ovary syndrome, cystic mastitis, obesity and infertility.

Source (edited): "http://en.wikipedia.org/wiki/SAHA_syndrome"

SCORAD

SCORAD ("SCORing Atopic Dermatitis") is a clinical tool for assessing the severity (i.e. extent, intensity) of atopic dermatitis as objectively as possible.

It was developed by the European Task Force on Atopic Dermatitis in 1993.

Source (edited): "http://en.wikipedia.org/wiki/SCORAD"

Scalp dysesthesia

Scalp dysesthesia is a cutaneous condition characterised by pain and burning sensations without objective physical examination findings.

Source (edited): "http://en.wikipedia.org/wiki/Scalp_dysesthesia"

Scalp pruritus

Scalp pruritus is an itchiness of the scalp, particularly common in elderly persons.

Source (edited): "http://en.wikipedia.org/wiki/Scalp_pruritus"

Scar sarcoid

Scar sarcoid (also known as "Sarcoidosis in scars") is a cutaneous condition characterized by infiltration and elevation of tattoos and old flat scars due to sarcoidosis.

Source (edited): "http://en.wikipedia.org/wiki/Scar_sarcoid"

Schamberg disease

Schamberg Disease, (also known as "Progressive pigmentary dermatosis of Schamberg," "Purpura pigmentosa progressiva," and "Schamberg's purpura") is a chronic discoloration of the skin found in people of all ages, usually affecting the legs. It slowly spreads throughout the body, and is most common in males. It is named after Jay Frank Schamberg, who described it in 1901.

Definition

Schamberg's disease, or progressive pigmented purpuric dermatitis, is a chronic discoloration of the skin which usually affects the legs and often spreads slowly. This disease is more common in males and may occur at any age from childhood onward.

Cause

Schamberg's disease is caused by leaky blood vessels near the surface of the skin, capillaries, which allow red blood cells to slip through into the skin. The red blood cells in the skin then fall apart and release their iron which causes a rust color, this accounts for the orange tint of the rash.

Symptoms

The lesions are most frequent on the lower limbs, but may occur anywhere on the body, including the hands. They may vary in number. They consist of irregular patches of orange or brown pigmentation due to hemosiderin (iron), with characteristic "cayenne pepper" spots appearing within and at the edge of old lesions. There are usually no symptoms, although there may be some slight itching. The eruption may persist for many years. The pattern of the eruption changes, with slow extension and often some clearing of the original lesions.

Treatment

There is no cure for Schamberg's disease; however, the itching can be controlled by a cortisone cream and Colchicine treatment has been successfully conducted, preventing recurrence of the symptoms.

Source (edited): "http://en.wikipedia.org/wiki/Schamberg_disease"

Schöpf–Schulz–Passarge syndrome

Schöpf–Schulz–Passarge syndrome (also known as "Eyelid cysts, palmoplantar keratoderma, hypodontia, and hypotrichosis") is an autosomal recessive condition with diffuse symmetric palmoplantar keratoderma, with the palmoplantar keratoderma and fragility of the nails beginning around age 12.

It was characterized in 1971.

It has been associated with WNT10A.

Source (edited): "http://en.wikipedia.org/wiki/Sch%C3%B6pf%E2%80%93Schulz%E2%80%93Passarge_syndrome"

Sciatic nerve injury

Sciatic nerve injury may occur from improperly performed injections into the buttock, and may result in sensory loss.

Source (edited): "http://en.wikipedia.org/wiki/Sciatic_nerve_injury"

Sclerema neonatorum

Sclerema neonatorum is a rare a severe skin condition that is characterized by inflammation of the underlying subcutaneous fat.

Source (edited): "http://en.wikipedia.org/wiki/Sclerema_neonatorum"

Scleroderma-like reaction to taxanes

Scleroderma-like reaction to taxanes may occur in patients treated with docetaxel or paclitaxel, characterized by an acute, diffuse, infiltrated edema of the extremities and head.

Source (edited): "http://en.wikipedia.org/wiki/Scleroderma-like_reaction_to_taxanes"

Sclerosing lipogranuloma

Sclerosing lipogranuloma (also known as a "Paraffinoma") is a skin condition characterized by a granulomatous and fibrotic reaction that occurs in the subcutaneous fat from the injection of silicone or mineral oils.

Source (edited): "http://en.wikipedia.org/wiki/Sclerosing_lipogranuloma"

Sclerosing lymphangiitis

Sclerosing lymphangiitis is a skin condition characterized by a cordlike structure encircling the coronal sulcus of the penis, or running the length of the shaft, that has been attributed to trauma during vigorous sexual play.

Source (edited): "http://en.wikipedia.org/wiki/Sclerosing_lymphangiitis"

Sea-blue histiocytosis

Sea-blue histiocytosis is a cutaneous condition that may occur as a familial inherited syndrome or as an acquired secondary or systemic infiltrative process.

Causes

It can be associated with the gene APOE.

It can also be acquired. Sea-blue histiocyte syndrome is seen in patients receiving fat emulsion as a part of long-term parenteral nutrition (TPN) for intestinal failure.

Pathophysiology and presentation

The high lipid content in the blood leads to excessive cytoplasm loading of lipids within histiocytes.

The subsequent incomplete degradation of these lipids leads to the formation of cytoplasmic lipid pigments.

High lipid content may also cause membrane abnormality of the hemopoietic cells which is recognized by macrophages and therefore, increased accumulation within the bone marrow.

These lipid laden histiocytes appear blue with May-Giemsa/PAS stain hence the name of Sea-Blue Histocyte Syndrome. Sea-blue histiocytosis is also seen in lipid disorders.

Source (edited): "http://en.wikipedia.org/wiki/Sea-blue_histiocytosis"

Seborrheic-like psoriasis

Seborrheic-like psoriasis (also known as "Sebopsoriasis," and "Seborrhiasis") is a skin condition characterized by psoriasis with an overlaping seborrheic dermatitis.

Source (edited): "http://en.wikipedia.org/wiki/Seborrheic-like_psoriasis"

Secondary cutaneous CD30+ large-cell lymphoma

Secondary cutaneous CD30+ large-cell lymphoma is a cutaneous condition that may arise in cases of mycosis fungoides, and in patients with lymphomatoid papulosis.

Source (edited): "http://en.wikipedia.org/wiki/Secondary_cutaneous_CD30%2B_large-cell_lymphoma"

Secondary cutaneous amyloidosis

Secondary cutaneous amyloidosis is a skin condition that occurs following PUVA therapy and in benign and malignant cutaneous neoplasms in which deopsits of amyloid may be found.

Source (edited): "http://en.wikipedia.org/wiki/Secondary_cutaneous_amyloidosis"

Secondary lymphedema

Secondary lymphedema is a condition characterized by swelling of the soft tissues in which an excessive amount of lymph has accumulated, and is caused by certain malignant diseases such as Hodgkin's disease and Kaposi sarcoma.

Source (edited): "http://en.wikipedia.org/wiki/Secondary_lymphedema"

Secondary systemic amyloidosis

Secondary systemic amyloidosis is a condition that involves the adrenal gland, liver, spleen, and kidney as a result of amyloid deposition due to a chronic disease such as Behçet's disease, ulcerative colitis, etc.

Source (edited): "http://en.wikipedia.org/wiki/Secondary_systemic_amyloidosis"

Self-healing juvenile cutaneous mucinosis

Self-healing juvenile cutaneous mucinosis is a skin condition caused by fibroblasts producing abnormally large amounts of mucopolysaccharides, and os characterized by the sudden onset of skin lesions and polyarthritis.

Source (edited): "http://en.wikipedia.org/wiki/Self-healing_juvenile_cutaneous_mucinosis"

Self-healing papular mucinosis

Self-healing papular mucinosis is a skin condition caused by fibroblasts producing abnormally large amounts of mucopolysaccharides, and may present in adult and juvenile forms. The juvenile variant is also called self-healing juvenile cutaneous mucinosis.

Source (edited): "http://en.wikipedia.org/wiki/Self-healing_papular_mucinosis"

Septal panniculitis

Septal panniculitis is a condition of the subcutaneous fat affecting the layer of adipose tissue that lies between the dermis and underlying fascia, of which there are two forms: acute erythema nodosum and chronic erythema nodosum.

Source (edited): "http://en.wikipedia.org/wiki/Septal_panniculitis"

Serum sickness-like reaction

Serum sickness-like reactions refer to adverse reactions that have similar symptoms to serum sickness, but in which immune complexes are not found.

Pathogenesis

Serum sickness-like reaction is named for its clinical similarity to serum sickness, in which immune complexes are deposited in the skin, joints, and other organs. True serum sickness, a type III hypersensitivity reaction, results in fever, lymphadenopathy, arthralgias,cutaneous eruptions, gastrointestinal disturbances, proteinuria,and significant decreases in serum complement levels; it was originally described after patients were infused with equine immunoglobulins.

In contrast, serum sickness-like reactions are specific drug reactions that are not associated with circulating immune complexes.

Although the exact pathogenesis is poorly understood,serum sickness-like reactions are thought to originate from an abnormal inflammatory reaction that occurs in response to defective metabolism of drug byproducts generated during pharmacologic therapy; the metabolic flaw could be a maternally-inherited trait. In vivo hepatic drug biotransformation studies have shown greater lymphocyte killing in subjects with a known history of serum sickness-like reactions than in control subjects.

Diagnosis

The reaction generally includes a constellation of fever; urticarial polycyclic wheals with central clearing on the trunk, extremities, face, and lateral borders of the hands and feet; oral edema without mucosal involvement; lymphadenopathy; arthralgias; myalgias; and mild proteinuria. Case reports have noted the absence of fever in serum sickness-like reactions to amoxicillin. Laboratory abnormalities include normal or mild decreases in serum C3, C4, and CH50 levels, and mild proteinuria, all of which were identified in our patient.1,3-5 In contrast to true serum sickness, renal and hepatic involvementis rare. Significant decreases in serum C3, C4, and CH50, reported in the literature for true serum sickness, are rarely described in serum sickness-like reaction.

Causes

Agents that have been implicated in serum sickness-like reactions include cefaclor, amoxicillin, sulfonamides, tetracyclines,ciprofloxacin, nonsteroidal anti-inflammatory drugs, barbiturates, carbamazepine, propranolol, thiouracil, and allopurinol. Metabolites of these drugs might bind with tissue proteins inappropriately, eliciting an acute inflammatory response that typically develops 7–14 days after initiation of the offending agent.

Management

Serum sickness-like reaction is an acute self-limited reaction with an ultimately favorable outcome. Treatment is typically symptomatic, but hospitalization may be required for severe cases. While optimal treatment strategies for serum sickness-like reactions are not clearly defined in the literature, discontinuation of the suspected agent combined with use of antihistamines and corticosteroids for symptom control is an appropriate therapeutic route. Case reports have shown that treatment with prednisone, 60 mg daily, and high doses of H1 and H2 antihistamines help resolve the arthralgias and myalgias within 24 hours and the remaining symptoms within 48–72 hours

Source (edited): "http://en.wikipedia.org/wiki/Serum_sickness-like_reaction"

Silica granuloma

Silica granulomas are a skin condition which may be caused by automobile and other types of accidents which produces tattooing of dirt (silicon dioxide) into the skin that then induces the granuloma formation.

Source (edited): "http://en.wikipedia.org/wiki/Silica_granuloma"

Silicone granuloma

Silicone granulomas are a skin condition that occur as a reaction to liquid silicones, and are characterized by the formation of nodules.

Source (edited): "http://en.wikipedia.org/wiki/Silicone_granuloma"

Small-sized congenital nevocytic nevus

Small-sized congenital nevocytic nevus is a cutaneous condition characterized by a nevus, generally defined as having a diameter less than 2cm.
Source (edited): "http://en.wikipedia.org/wiki/Small-sized_congenital_nevocytic_nevus"

Small plaque parapsoriasis

Small plaque parapsoriasis (also known as **chronic superficial dermatitis**) characteristically occurs with skin lesions that are round, oval, discrete patches or thin plaques, mainly on the trunk.
Source (edited): "http://en.wikipedia.org/wiki/Small_plaque_parapsoriasis"

Smooth tongue

Smooth tongue (also known as "Atrophic glossitis," "Bald tongue," "Hunter glossitis," and "Moeller glossitis") is a condition characterized by a smooth glossy tongue that is often tender/painful.
Source (edited): "http://en.wikipedia.org/wiki/Smooth_tongue"

Solar erythema

Solar erythema is a skin condition characterized by redness of the skin following exposure to ultraviolet light, not to be confused with sunburn.
Source (edited): "http://en.wikipedia.org/wiki/Solar_erythema"

Solar purpura

Solar purpura (also known as "Actinic purpura," and "Senile purpura") is a skin condition characterized by large, sharply outlined, 1- to 5-cm, dark purplish-red ecchymoses appearing on the dorsa of the forearms and less often the hands.

The condition is most common in elderly white persons. It is caused by sun-induced damage to the connective tissue of the skin.

No treatment is necessary. The lesions typically fade over a period of up to 3 weeks.
Source (edited): "http://en.wikipedia.org/wiki/Solar_purpura"

Spitz nevus

A **Spitz nevus** (also known as an "Epithelioid and spindle-cell nevus," "Benign juvenile melanoma", and "Spitz's juvenile melanoma") is a benign melanocytic nevus, a type of skin lesion, affecting the epidermis and dermis.

Spitz nevus is also known as spindle and epithelioid cell nevus and juvenile melanoma. The latter term is generally no longer used as it is misleading: it is not a melanoma, it is a benign lesion; it can also occur in adults, not only in children.

The lesion is named after Dr.Sophie Spitz, the pathologist who originally described it in 1948.

Epidemiology

Spitz nevi are uncommon. Their annual incidence was estimated in a coastal population of sub-tropical Queensland to be 1.4 cases per 100,000 people. For comparison, the annual incidence of melanoma in the same population, which is high by world standards is 25.4 cases per 100,000 people.

Whilst they are most commonly found on people in their first two decades of life, the age range for people with Spitz nevi is from six months to 71 years, with a mean age of twenty-two years and a median age of nineteen years.

Causes

The cause of Spitz nevi is not yet known. There is an association with sunburn, but causation is not established. Genetic studies of Spitz nevi have shown that most cells have the normal number of chromosomes, however a minority (25%) of cells have been shown to contain extra copies of parts of some chromosomes, such as the short arm of chromosome 11 (11p).
Source (edited): "http://en.wikipedia.org/wiki/Spitz_nevus"

Stasis dermatitis

Stasis dermatitis (also known as "Congestion eczema," "Gravitational dermatitis," "Gravitational eczema," "Stasis eczema," and "Varicose eczema") refers to the skin changes that occur in the leg as a result of "stasis" or blood pooling from insufficient venous return; the alternative name of **varicose eczema** comes from a common cause of this being varicose veins.

Insufficient venous return results in increased pressure in the capillaries with the result that both fluid and cells may "leak" out of the capillaries. This results in red cells breaking down, with iron containing hemosiderin possibly contributing to the pathology of this entity.

Symptoms

- The skin appears thin, brown and tissue-like, with possible skin lesions (macule or patches), red spots, superficial skin irritation and/or darkening and/or thickening of the skin at the ankles or legs.
- The skin may be weakened and ulcerate in areas.
- Legs, ankles, or other areas may be swollen.
- Open sores, ulcers
- Itching and/or leg pains

The cracks and poor skin condition of this disorder predisposes for the entry of bacterial infection causing spreading cellulitis infection in the leg. If the skin condition deteriorates further and breaks down, a venous ulcer (also known as statis ulcer) may form.

Treatment

Treatment may consist of topical applications of steroid based creams and the use of compression stockings to help force the underlying buildup of fluids back out of the lower leg or sequential gradient pump therapy. Sequential Gradient Pump Therapy has been used over 30 years throughout the world.

Source (edited): "http://en.wikipedia.org/wiki/Stasis_dermatitis"

Steroid acne

Steroid acne is an adverse reaction to corticosteroids, and presents as small, firm follicular papules on the forehead, cheeks, and chest.

Source (edited): "http://en.wikipedia.org/wiki/Steroid_acne"

Steroid folliculitis

Steroid folliculitis occurs following administration of glucocorticoids or corticotropin.

Source (edited): "http://en.wikipedia.org/wiki/Steroid_folliculitis"

Stewart–Treves syndrome

Stewart-Treves syndrome refers to an angiosarcoma arising from chronic lymphedema (swelling due to lymphatic obstruction). It typically occurs as a complication of long-lasting lymphedema of the arm after mastectomy and/or radiotherapy for breast cancer. It can rarely occur on the leg. The prognosis, even with wide surgical excision and subsequent radiotherapy, is poor.

Angiosarcoma is a malignant tumor of vascular origin. It accounts for less than 1% of all sarcomas and is usually located in the skin, breast, liver, and soft tissue.

Source (edited): "http://en.wikipedia.org/wiki/Stewart%E2%80%93Treves_syndrome"

Striae distensae

Striae distensae are depressed lines or bands of thin reddened skin, which later become white, smooth, shiny, and depressed, occurring in response to changes in weight or muscle mass and skin tension. They are commonly referred to as stretch marks.

Treatment

Fractional Photothermolysis can be used to treat Striae Distensae.

Source (edited): "http://en.wikipedia.org/wiki/Striae_distensae"

Striae gravidarum

Striae gravidarum are a cutaneous condition characterized by stretch marks (Striae distensae) on the abdomen during and following pregnancy.

Source (edited): "http://en.wikipedia.org/wiki/Striae_gravidarum"

Striate keratoderma

Striate keratodermas are a group of autosomal dominant palmoplantar keratodermas with streaking hyperkeratosis involving the finders and extending onto the palm of the hand.
Source (edited): "http://en.wikipedia.org/wiki/Striate_keratoderma"

Striate palmoplantar keratoderma

Striate palmoplantar keratoderma (also known as "Acral keratoderma," "Brünauer-Fuhs-Siemens type of palmoplantar keratoderma," "Focal nonepidermolytic palmoplantar keratoderma," "Keratosis palmoplantaris varians," "Palmoplantar keratoderma areata," "Palmoplantar keratoderma striata," "Wachter keratoderma," and "Wachters palmoplantar keratoderma") is a cutaneous condition, an autosomal dominant keratoderma principally involving the soles with onset in infancy or the first few years of life.

- Type 1: 148700: DSG1
- Type 2: 612908: DSP
- Type 3: 607654: KRT1

Source (edited): "http://en.wikipedia.org/wiki/Striate_palmoplantar_keratoderma"

Subacute cutaneous lupus erythematosus

Subacute cutaneous lupus erythematosus is a clinically distinct subset of cases of lupus erythematosus that is most often present in white women aged 15 to 40, consisting of skin lesions that are scaly and evolve as polycyclic annular lesions or psoriasiform plaques.

Characteristically the lesions appear in sun-exposed areas such as the vee of the neckline or the forearms, but not the face. It may be brought on by sun-sensitizing medications, but is usually associated with autoimmune disorders such as rheumatoid arthritis and Sjögren's syndrome.

Treatment generally involves sun avoidance/protection and topical corticosteroids.

Lesions of SCLE may have an annular configuration, with raised red borders and central clearing.
Source (edited): "http://en.wikipedia.org/wiki/Subacute_cutaneous_lupus_erythematosus"

Subcorneal pustular dermatosis

Subcorneal pustular dermatosis (also known as "Sneddon–Wilkinson disease") is skin condition that is a rare, chronic, recurrent, pustular eruption characterized histopathologically by subcorneal pustules that contain abundant neutrophils.
Source (edited): "http://en.wikipedia.org/wiki/Subcorneal_pustular_dermatosis"

Subcutaneous T-cell lymphoma

Subcutaneous T-cell lymphoma (also known as a "Panniculitis-like T-cell lymphoma") is a cutaneous condition that most commonly presents in young adults, and is characterized by subcutaneous nodules.

Classification

Subcutaneous panniculitis-like T-cell lymphoma, is a subtype of Peripheral T-cell lymphoma. Peripheral T-cell lymphoma (PTCL) is defined as a diverse group of aggressive lymphomas that develop from mature-stage white blood cells called T-cells and natural killer cells (NK cells) (see figure for an overview of PTCL subtypes). PTCL is a type of non-Hodgkin's lymphoma (NHL). NHL affects two particular types of white blood cells: B-cells and T-cells. PTCL specifically affects T-cells, and results when T-cells develop and grow abnormally.

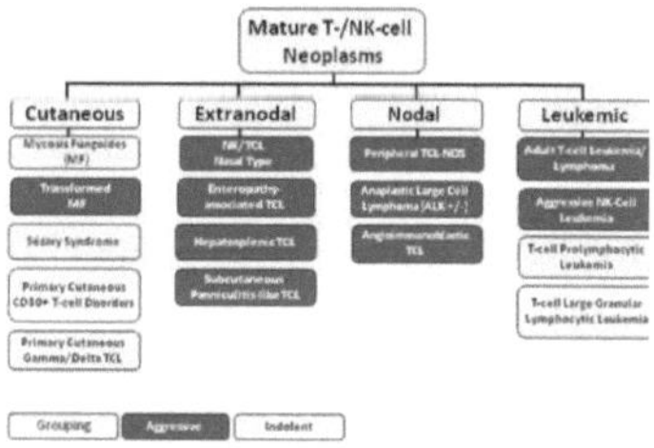

Figure 1 (*adapted from Rodriguez J, et al. Crit Rev Oncol Hematol. 2008*)

Subcutaneous Panniculitis-like T-cell Lymphoma is a rare type of lymphoma that infiltrates the subcutaneous fat but does not involve the skin. There are two subtypes – alpha-beta and gamma-delta.

Patients with the gamma-delta subtype have a more aggressive clinical course.

Treatment

Currently Subcutaneous Panniculitis-like T-cell Lymphoma, being a PTCL subtype, is treated similarly to B-cell lymphomas. However, in recent years, scientists have developed techniques to better recognize the different types of lymphomas, such as PTCL. It is now understood that PTCL behaves differently from B-cell lymphomas and therapies are being developed that specifically target these types of lymphoma. Currently, however, there are no therapies approved by the U.S. Food and Drug Administration (FDA) specifically for PTCL. Anthracycline-containing chemotherapy regimens are commonly offered as the initial therapy. Some patients may receive a stem cell transplant. Novel approaches to the treatment of PTCL in the relapsed or refractory setting are under investigation.

Research

Pralatrexate is one compound currently under investigations for the treatment of PTCL. For information please consult the US clinical trials database (http://www.clinicaltrials.gov).
Source (edited): "http://en.wikipedia.org/wiki/Subcutaneous_T-cell_lymphoma"

Subcutaneous fat necrosis of the newborn

Subcutaneous fat necrosis of the newborn (SCFN or SFN) is a rare form of lobular panniculitis occurring in newborns that is usually self-remitting and non-recurring. Proposed causes include perinatal stress, local trauma, hypoxia and hypothermia, though the exact cause is unknown. It has been suggested that the brown fat seen in newborns is more sensitive to hypoxic injury than fat seen in adults, and that such hypoxia, usually in the context of a complicated birth, leads to the fat necrosis. Complications can include hypercalcemia, hyperlipidemia and thrombocytopenia, and can present months after the onset of SCFN symptoms..
Source (edited): "http://en.wikipedia.org/wiki/Subcutaneous_fat_necrosis_of_the_newborn"

Subcutaneous granuloma annulare

Subcutaneous granuloma annulare (also known as "Deep granuloma annulare," and "Pseudorheumatoid nodule") is a skin condition of unknown cause, most commonly affecting children, with boys affected twice as commonly as girls, characterized by skin lesions most often on the lower legs.
Source (edited): "http://en.wikipedia.org/wiki/Subcutaneous_granuloma_annulare"

Subcutaneous sarcoidosis

Subcutaneous sarcoidosis (also known as "Darier–Roussy disease" and "Darier-Roussy sarcoid") is a cutaneous condition characterized by numerous 0.5- to 0.3-cm deep-seated nodules on the trunk and extremities.
Source (edited): "http://en.wikipedia.org/wiki/Subcutaneous_sarcoidosis"

Subepidermal calcified nodule

Subepidermal calcified nodule (also known as a "Solitary congenital nodular calcification," and "Winer's nodular calcinosis") is a cutaneous condition characterized by calcification of the skin resulting from the deposition of calcium and phosphorus, occurring most frequently as one or a few skin lesions on the scalp or face of children.
Source (edited): "http://en.wikipedia.org/wiki/Subepidermal_calcified_nodule"

Sulfonamide hypersensitivity syndrome

Sulfonamide hypersensitivity syndrome is similar to anticonvulsant hypersensitivity syndrome, but the onset is often sooner in the treatment course, generally after 7-14 days of therapy.

It is considered immune-mediated.
Source (edited): "http://en.wikipedia.org/wiki/Sulfonamide_hypersensitivity_syndrome"

Superficial thrombophlebitis

Superficial thrombophlebitis is an inflammation and thrombosis of superficial veins which presents as a painful induration with erythema, often in a linear or branching configuration forming cords.

Source (edited): "http://en.wikipedia.org/wiki/Superficial_thrombophlebitis"

Tar melanosis

Tar melanosis (also known as "Melanodermatitis toxica lichenoides") is an occupational dermatosis that occurs among tar handlers after several years' exposure, characterized by a severe widespread itching that is soon followed by the appearance of reticular pigmentation, telangiectases, and a shiny appearance of the skin.

Source (edited): "http://en.wikipedia.org/wiki/Tar_melanosis"

Texier's disease

Texier's disease is a pseudosclerodermatous reaction that occurs after injection with vitamin K, a subcutaneous sclerosis with or without fasciitis that lasts several years.

Source (edited): "http://en.wikipedia.org/wiki/Texier%27s_disease"

Thymoma with immunodeficiency

Thymoma with immunodeficiency (also known as "Good syndrome") is a condition that occurs in adults in whom hypogammaglobulinemia, deficient cell-mediated immunity, and benign thymoma may develop almost simultaneously.

Source (edited): "http://en.wikipedia.org/wiki/Thymoma_with_immunodeficiency"

Titanium metallic discoloration

Titanium metallic discoloration has been reported to have occurred with titanium-containing ointment causing papules on the penis of a patient. Titanium screws used for orthopedic procedures, if they come in close proximity to the skin, can also causes cutaneous blue-black hyperpigmentation.

Source (edited): "http://en.wikipedia.org/wiki/Titanium_metallic_discoloration"

Transient erythroporphyria of infancy

Transient erythroporphyria of infancy (also known as "Purpuric phototherapy-induced eruption") is a cutaneous condition reported in infants exposed to blue lights for the treatment of indirect hyperbilirubinemia characterized by marked purpura in skin exposed to the UV light.

Source (edited): "http://en.wikipedia.org/wiki/Transient_erythroporphyria_of_infancy"

Transient neonatal pustular melanosis

Transient neonatal pustular melanosis (also known as "Transient neonatal pustulosis", and "Lentigines neonatorum") is a cutaneous condition that presents at birth with 1- to 3-mm flaccid, superficial fragile pustules, some of which may have already resolved in utero, leaving pigmented macules.

Source (edited): "http://en.wikipedia.org/wiki/Transient_neonatal_pustular_melanosis"

Traumatic calcinosis cutis

Traumatic calcinosis cutis is a cutaneous condition characterized by calcification of the skin resulting from the deposition of calcium and phosphorus often resulting from occupational exposure, as in cases reported in oil-field workers and coal miners.

Source (edited): "http://en.wikipedia.org/wiki/Traumatic_calcinosis_cutis"

Traumatic panniculitis

Traumatic panniculitis is a skin condition characterized by inflammation and necrosis of the subcutaneous fat following accidental trauma to the skin.

Source (edited): "http://en.wikipedia.org/wiki/Traumatic_panniculitis"

Traumatic purpura

Traumatic purpura is a skin condition resulting from trauma which produces ecchymoses of bizarre shapes suggestive of abuse.

Source (edited): "http://en.wikipedia.org/wiki/Traumatic_purpura"

Trigeminal trophic lesion

Trigeminal trophic lesions (also known as "Trigeminal trophic syndrome") are a cutaneous condition caused by the interruption of peripheral or central sensory pathways of the trigeminal nerve that result in a slowly enlarging, uninflammed ulcer on the cheek beside the ala nasi.

Source (edited): "http://en.wikipedia.org/wiki/Trigeminal_trophic_lesion"

Tropical acne

Tropical acne is unusually severe acne occurring in the tropics during seasons when the weather is hot and humid.

Source (edited): "http://en.wikipedia.org/wiki/Tropical_acne"

Tropical anhidrotic asthenia

Tropical anhidrotic asthenia is a skin condition, a rare form of miliaria, with long-lasting poral occlusion, which produces anhidrosis and heat retention.

Source (edited): "http://en.wikipedia.org/wiki/Tropical_anhidrotic_asthenia"

Tropical immersion foot

Tropical immersion foot (also known as "Paddy foot", and "Paddy-field foot") is a skin condition of the feet seen after continuous immersion of the feet in water or mud of temperature above 22 degrees Celsius for two to ten days.

Source (edited): "http://en.wikipedia.org/wiki/Tropical_immersion_foot"

Trumpeter's wart

A **trumpeter's wart** is a cutaneous condition characterized by a firm, fibrous, hyperkeratotic nodule on the upper lip of a trumpet player.

Source (edited): "http://en.wikipedia.org/wiki/Trumpeter%27s_wart"

Tumid lupus erythematosus

Tumid lupus erythematosus (also known as "lupus erythematosus tumidus") is a rare, but distinctive entity in which patients present with edematous erythematous plaques, usually on the trunk.

Lupus erythematosus tumidus (LET) was reported by Henri Gougerot and Burnier R. in 1930. It is a photosensitive skin disorder, a different subtype of cutaneous lupus erythematosus (CLE) from discoid lupus erythematosus (DLE) or subacute CLE (SCLE). LET is usually found on sun-exposed areas of the body. Skin lesions are edematous, urticarialike annular papules and plaques. Topical corticosteroids are not effective as treatment for LET, but many will respond to chloroquine. LET resolves with normal skin, no residual scarring, no hyperpigmentation or hypopigmentation. Cigarette smokers who have LET may not respond very well to chloroquine.

It has been suggested that it is equivalent to Jessner lymphocytic infiltrate of the skin.

Source (edited): "http://en.wikipedia.org/wiki/Tumid_lupus_erythematosus"

Tumoral calcinosis

Tumoral calcinosis is a skin condition characterized by calcification of a pre-existing skin tumor (the tumor can be either benign such as a pilomatrixoma or malignant such as a basal cell carcinoma); it presents as large subcutaneous masses. The original tumor may or may not disappear leaving behind a calcified nodule that may eventually ossify (turn to bone).

Source (edited): "http://en.wikipedia.org/wiki/Tumoral_calcinosis"

Tyrosinemia type II

Tyrosinemia type II (also known as "Oculocutaneous tyrosinemia," and "Richner-Hanhart syndrome") is an autosomal recessive condition with onset between ages 2 and 4 years, when painful circumscribed callosities develop on the pressure points of the palm and sole.

Pathophysiology

Type II tyrosinemia is caused by a deficiency of the enzyme tyrosine aminotransferase (EC 2.6.1.5), encoded by the gene *TAT*. Tyrosine aminotransferase is the first in a series of five enzymes that converts tyrosine to smaller molecules, which are excreted by the kidneys or used in reactions that produce energy. This form of the disorder can affect the eyes, skin, and mental development. Symptoms often begin in early childhood and include excessive tearing, abnormal sensitivity to light (photophobia), eye pain and redness, and painful skin lesions on the palms and soles. About half of individuals with type II tyrosinemia are also mentally challenged. Type II tyrosinemia occurs in fewer than 1 in 250,000 individuals.

Source (edited): "http://en.wikipedia.org/wiki/Tyrosinemia_type_II"

Ulcerative lichen planus

Ulcerative lichen planus is a rare variant of lichen planus presenting with chronic, painful bullae and ulceration of the feet, often with cicatricial sequelae evident.

Source (edited): "http://en.wikipedia.org/wiki/Ulcerative_lichen_planus"

Ulcerative sarcoidosis

Ulcerative sarcoidosis is a cutaneous condition affecting roughly 5% of people with sarcoidosis.

Source (edited): "http://en.wikipedia.org/wiki/Ulcerative_sarcoidosis"

Ullrich disease

Ullrich disease is a genetic extracellular matrix diseases of the skin characterized by puffy skin.

Source (edited): "http://en.wikipedia.org/wiki/Ullrich_disease"

Uranium dermatosis

Uranium dermatosis is a cutaneous condition characterized by an irritant contact dermatitis and skin burns due to exposure to uranium.

Source (edited): "http://en.wikipedia.org/wiki/Uranium_dermatosis"

Uremic pruritus

Uremic pruritus (also known as "Renal pruritus") is caused by chronic renal failure and is the most common internal systemic cause of pruritus.

Pathogenesis of Uremic Pruritus

The cause of uremic pruritus is not fully

clarified. Oveactivity of type 1 T helper cells (TH1) has been demonstrated in uremic pruritus. Furthermore, serum levels of interleukin-2, a cytokine produced by TH1 cells, have been demonstrated to be higher in dialysis patients with itch compared to dialysis patients without itch. This cytokine has a well-documented role in induction of pruritus. Other proposed contributors to the pathogenesis of uremic pruritus include anemia or other manifestation of erythropoietin deficiency, inadequate dialysis, histamine release from skin mast cells, skin dryness, secondary hyperparathyroidism, hyperphosphatemia with increased calcium phosphate deposition in the skin and alterations in the endogenous opioidergic system with overexpression of opioid μ-receptors.

Treatment of Uremic Pruritus

Therapeutic modalities and medications that target TH1 cells and inhibit production of interleukin-2 such as ultraviolet B phototherapy, tacrolimus and thalidomide have been demonstrated to be effective in treatment of uremic pruritus. Other therapeutic options include gabapentin, opoiod antagonists such as naltrexone, topical capsaicin, emollients, treating anemia of chronic kidney disease with erythropoietin, optimizing dialysis dose and antihistamines.
Source (edited): "http://en.wikipedia.org/wiki/Uremic_pruritus"

Urticarial erythema multiforme

Urticarial erythema multiforme is an unusual reaction virtually always associated with antibiotic ingestions, characterized by skin lesions that consist of urticarial papules and plaques, some of which clear centrally forming annular lesions, but with no true urticarial lesions.
Source (edited): "http://en.wikipedia.org/wiki/Urticarial_erythema_multiforme"

Venous insufficiency ulceration

Venous insufficiency ulceration, as well as stasis dermatitis, is a skin condition that results from increased pressure in the venous system of the lower leg.
Source (edited): "http://en.wikipedia.org/wiki/Venous_insufficiency_ulceration"

Verrucous lupus erythematosus

Verrucous lupus erythematosus (also known as "Hypertrophic lupus erythematosus") presents with non-puritic papulonodular lesions on the arms and hands, resembling keratoacanthoma or hypertropic lichen planus.
Source (edited): "http://en.wikipedia.org/wiki/Verrucous_lupus_erythematosus"

Vibratory angioedema

Vibratory angioedema is a form of physical urticaria that may be an inherited autosomal dominant trait, or may be acquired after prolonged occupational vibration exposure.
Source (edited): "http://en.wikipedia.org/wiki/Vibratory_angioedema"

Vitamin K reaction

Vitamin K reactions occur after injection with vitamin K, and there are two patterns of presentation, (1) a reaction may occur several days to 2 weeks after inection with skin lesions that are pruritic, red patches and plaques that can deep-seated, involving the dermis and subcutaneous tissue, or (2) with subcutaneous sclerosis with or without fasciitis, that appears at the site of injection many months after treatment. The latter pseudosclerodermatous reaction has been termed Texier's disease and lasts several years.
Source (edited): "http://en.wikipedia.org/wiki/Vitamin_K_reaction"

Vohwinkel syndrome

Vohwinkel syndome (also known as "Keratoderma hereditaria mutilans," "Keratoma hereditaria mutilans," "Mutilating keratoderma of Vohwinkel", "Mutilating palmoplantar keratoderma") is a diffuse autosomal dominant keratoderma with onset in early infancy characterized by a honeycombed keratoderma involving the palmoplantar surfaces. Mild to moderate sensorineural hearing loss is often associated.

It has been associated with GJB2.

It was characterized in 1929.

Source (edited): "http://en.wikipedia.org/wiki/Vohwinkel_syndrome"

Waldenström hyperglobulinemic purpura

Waldenström hyperglobulinemic purpura (also known as "Purpura hyperglobulinemica") is a skin condition that presents with episodic showers of petechiae (small red or purple spots) occurring on all parts of the body, most profusely on the lower extremities.

Source (edited): "http://en.wikipedia.org/wiki/Waldenstr%C3%B6m_hyperglobulinemic_purpura"

Warm water immersion foot

Warm water immersion foot is a skin condition of the feet that results after exposure to warm, wet conditions for 48 hours or more, and is characterized by maceration, blanching, and wrinkling of the soles and sides of the feet.

Source (edited): "http://en.wikipedia.org/wiki/Warm_water_immersion_foot"

Waxy skin

Waxy skin is a cutaneous condition observed in roughly 50% of diabetic patients with longstanding disease.

Source (edited): "http://en.wikipedia.org/wiki/Waxy_skin"

Weathering nodule of ear

Weathering nodules of ear is a cutaneous condition seen on the helices of the ears of Caucasian men who have a history of significant cumulative sun exposure.

Source (edited): "http://en.wikipedia.org/wiki/Weathering_nodule_of_ear"

Weber–Christian disease

Weber–Christian disease (also known as "Relapsing febrile non-suppurative panniculitis") is a cutaneous condition characterized by recurrent subcutaneous nodules that heal with depression of the overlying skin.

It is type of panniculitis.

Eponym

It is named for Frederick Parkes Weber and Henry Asbury Christian.

Source (edited): "http://en.wikipedia.org/wiki/Weber%E2%80%93Christian_disease"

Wende–Bauckus syndrome

Wende–Bauckus syndrome (also known as "Pegum syndrome") is a cutaneous condition characterized by tiny white macules on the trunk with confluence within flexures.

Source (edited): "http://en.wikipedia.org/wiki/Wende%E2%80%93Bauckus_syndrome"

Wrinkly skin syndrome

Wrinkly skin syndrome is a hereditary connective tissue disorder that is inherited in an autosomal recessive fashion.

Source (edited): "http://en.wikipedia.org/wiki/Wrinkly_skin_syndrome"

X-linked hyper-immunoglobulin M syndrome

X-linked hyper-immunoglobulin M syndrome is an inherited condition characterized by recurrent sinopulmonary and GI infections with pyogenic bacteria and opportunistic organisms, a disease which may have cutaneous manifestations including pyodermas extensive warts.

Source (edited): "http://en.wikipedia.org/wiki/X-linked_hyper-immunoglobulin_M_syndrome"

X-linked reticulate pigmentary disorder

X-linked reticulate pigmentary disorder (also known as "Familial cutaneous amyloidosis," "Partington amyloidosis," "Partington cutaneous amyloidosis," "Partington syndrome type II," "Reticulate pigmentary disorder", and "X-linked reticulate pigmentary disorder with systemic manifestations") is a cutaneous condition that has been described in adult women that had linear streaks of hyperpigmentation and in which male patients manifested a reticulated mottled brown pigmentation of the skin, which, on biopsy, demonstrated dermal deposits of amyloid.

The syndrome is also referred with the acronym **X-Linked-PDR** or even **XLPRD**.

It's a very rare disease, genetically determined, with a chronic course.

The gene responsible for the disease has not yet been identified. It is expected to be in the range of Xp21-Xp22.

It was characterized in 1981.

Presentation

Affected males develop generalized reticular hyper pigmentation in early childhood. Hair often looks bedraggled or brushed backwards, hanging low on the forehead.

Among the associated extracutaneous manifestations are described:

- Respiratory infections
- Dyskeratosis corneal photophobia
- Hypohidrosis with large deficit of thermoregulation
- Growth retardation
- Gastrointestinal disorders
- Kidney disease
- Kidney stones
- Urinary infections
- Webbed feet or hands
- Electrolyte imbalance
- Retinitis pigmentosa
- Lymphoedema
- Thyroid abnormalities

Each patient shows some of the symptoms listed above. Not every sick person will show all of the listed symptoms.

In females the disease is characterized by skin rashes linear hyper pigmentation following the Blaschko's lines, morphologically similar to stage 3 pigment incontinence. There are no systemic manifestations associated with XLPDR in females.

Source (edited): "http://en.wikipedia.org/wiki/X-linked_reticulate_pigmentary_disorder"

X-type histiocytosis

X-type histiocytoses are a clinically well-defined group of cutaneous syndromes characterized by infiltrates of Langerhans cells, as opposed to Non-X histiocytosis in which the infiltrates contain monocytes/macrophages. Conditions included in this group are:

- Congenital self-healing reticulohistiocytosis
- Langerhans cell histiocytosis

Source (edited): "http://en.wikipedia.org/wiki/X-type_histiocytosis"

Xanthoerythrodermia perstans

Xanthoerythrodermia perstans is a distinct variant of small-plaque parapsoriasis with lesions that are yellow in color.

Source (edited): "http://en.wikipedia.org/wiki/Xanthoerythrodermia_perstans"

Xanthoma diabeticorum

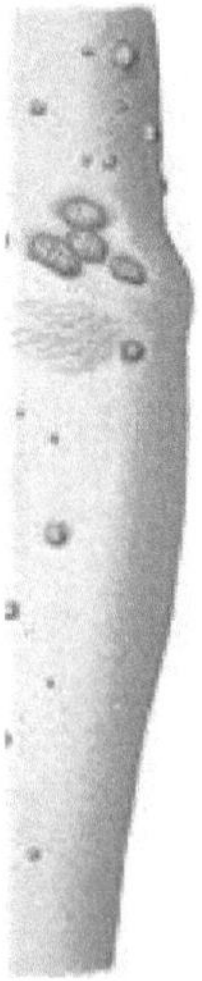
Xanthoma diabetacorum.

Xanthoma diabeticorum is a cutaneous condition that may result in young persons who are unresponsive to insulin.
Source (edited): "http://en.wikipedia.org/wiki/Xanthoma_diabeticorum"

Xanthoma disseminatum

Xanthoma disseminatum (also known as "Disseminated xanthosiderohistiocytosis" and "Montgomery syndrome") is a rare cutaneous condition that preferentially affects males in childhood, characterized by the insidious onset of small, yellow-red to brown papules and nodules that are discrete and disseminated.

It is a histiocytosis syndrome.
Source (edited): "http://en.wikipedia.org/wiki/Xanthoma_disseminatum"

Xanthoma striatum palmare

Xanthoma striatum palmare is a cutaneous condition characterized by xanthomas of the palmar creases which are almost diagnostic for dysbetalipoproteinemia.
Source (edited): "http://en.wikipedia.org/wiki/Xanthoma_striatum_palmare"

Xanthomatous biliary cirrhosis

Xanthomatous biliary cirrhosis (also known as "Obstructive liver disease") is a condition in which there is hyperlipoproteinemia due to liver disease resulting in plane xanthomas.
Source (edited): "http://en.wikipedia.org/wiki/Xanthomatous_biliary_cirrhosis"

Xerotic eczema

Xerotic eczema (also known as "Eczema craquelé", "Pruritus hiemalis", "Asteatotic eczema", "Winter itch", "Desiccation dermatitis," and "Winter eczema") is a form of eczema that is characterized by changes that occur when skin becomes abnormally dry, itchy, and cracked. Lower legs tend to be especially affected, although it can appear in the underarm area as well.

Xerotic eczema is common in elderly people, though it is not uncommon for people in their 20s. It can appear in red, bumpy, pimple-like irritations. Shaving can cause it to become inflamed.

Treatment

One way to treat xerotic eczema is to avoid scratching the affected area and to apply anti-itch or moisturizing lotion frequently.

A study published in 2005 found positive results when the affected area was soaked in water for twenty minutes and subsequently applying mid- to high-strength corticosteroid ointment.
Source (edited): "http://en.wikipedia.

org/wiki/Xerotic_eczema"

Yemenite deaf-blind hypopigmentation syndrome

Yemenite deaf-blind hypopigmentation syndrome is a condition caused by a mutation on the SRY-related HMG-box gene 10 (not SOX10).

It was characterized in 1990.

Some sources affirm *SOX10* involvement.

Source (edited): "http://en.wikipedia.org/wiki/Yemenite_deaf-blind_hypopigmentation_syndrome"

Zirconium granuloma

Zirconium granulomas are a skin condition characterized by a papular eruption involving the axillae, and are sometimes considered an allergic reaction to deodorant containing zirconium lactate.

Source (edited): "http://en.wikipedia.org/wiki/Zirconium_granuloma"